CONTENTS

Acknowledgements

With a full heart I should like to thank Bridget for getting me going, Alan for his kindness and friendship and Robert, from whom I learnt more than I could have imagined. I would also like to thank Barbara for her "pushiness" and for her great care; the spirit of Miss Basket at Upper Wyckam Manor and all the Gregorys - but special thanks to Anna for her love and support during difficult times (and also for being a fairy godmother!). My love and my gratitude go to many, through thick and especially thin, but most of all to Tom for being there, my midwife Ann Minter, who made all the difference, and to my publisher Ian Miller, for being so patient and making me laugh.

JANE DYE

AROMATHERAPY
FOR WOMEN & CHILDREN
Pregnancy and Childbirth

Index compiled by
Lyn Greenwood

SAFFRON WALDEN
THE C. W. DANIEL COMPANY LIMITED

For Josie

First published in Great Britain in 1992
by The C. W. Daniel Company Limited
1 Church Path, Saffron Walden
Essex, CB10 1JP, England

ISBN 0 85207 226 0

Designed by Peter Dolton
Produced in association with Book Production Consultants, Cambridge
Typeset by Cambridge Photosetting Services
Printed and bound by St Edmundsbury Press,
Bury St Edmunds, Suffolk

INTRODUCTION

......................❖......................

After several months study in therapeutic massage and sports injuries, learning about the countless benefits and the many healing properties of massage, correct exercise and the importance of a balanced diet and nutrition - I then heard about aromatherapy and the use of essential oils.

Double doors of delight, wonder and fascination were thrown open to me, as this was to be the beginning of a learning that makes sense to me in every single way.

Holistic aromatherapy, is essentially a natural therapy, and, if used with kowledge understanding and respect, can help to establish and maintain health and well being in a safe, non-toxic and non-habit forming way. It is a highly successful therapy for any stress related conditions and has the added bonus of boosting our own natural immunity and resources to combat all manner of ailments - from verrucas to bronchitis. Aromatherapy is also a deeply wonderful experience.

The role of all natural therapeutics is to encourage and stimulate these natural resources within us all, reducing dependence on chemical drugs where possible, with their sometimes unfortunate side effects, and to stimulate natural and effective response in a safe way, without causing additional imbalance to our systems. This is especially important when treating children and during pregnancy, when almost whatever you do, however you feel, affects not only you but also your child.

Of the many types of body contact therapies, massage is the most common, as most of us respond very deeply to touch, humans being essentially tactile beings. Some do prefer other associated therapies - such as homeopathy or acupuncture, although both can effectively complement aromatherapy. An aromatherapy massage makes the most effective use of essential oils, as massage can stimulate and relax muscles, improve circulation and encourage lymph flow, improve digestion and body function and aid waste elimination. Massage is a natural healing instinct within us all, for whenever pain or unease is felt, the involuntary action of rubbing the painful area, or even simply holding yourself or another, is the most immediate and natural of all impulses and often the most effective. Think of the healing power of a cuddle...

This book is not intended as a substitute for professional advice, but is a general guide to help with the more common conditions which holistic aromatherapy can effectively treat. However, if you have any doubt at all about the seriousness of some symptoms, seek specialist advice and treatment from your GP or a fully qualified aromatherapist. The book has been written with women, pregnancy and children in mind, but equally applies (for some conditions!) to all members of the family who will benefit from the countless therapeutic effects, along with the sheer pleasure of the therapy. Throughout the book, I have referred to the standard "he", as "she", not to exclude the boys, but because my daughter and I were so involved with the writing of this book, from conception onwards - so mothers of boys please forgive me, but the treatments given apply equally to both sexes, unless otherwise stated.

We are all travelling a miraculous journey, which began probably before actual conception - and along which we will pass only once. If pregnant, you and your baby need to make this time together as special and as safe as possible, for both of you. At many stages along the way, we all need some care and healing, whether it's a cuddle, a holiday, or treatment for something more serious - either by orthodox or complementary means. Both are valid and make sense, and both can and should complement each other, avoiding at all times, a "them and us" conflict.

Orthodox practicioners are becoming increasingly aware of the benefits of complementary/alternative medicine and that they are not all "wacky" – with no scientific basis. Likewise, alternative should always be complementary, with all sharing a common wish for patients, in whichever camp, to regain their ability to mobilise inner resources and faith in themselves, no matter what their religion or beliefs – to aid recovery and a feeling of their own responsibility and involvement.

Many trials are being conducted and reports gradually

being published on the scientific validity of this previously neglected area of therapy – so look out for continual updates on aromatherapy and the use of essential oils.

Aromatherapy can bring a smile both inside and out, and Mother Nature has given us the precious gift of our being able to share in some of her secrets - let us rediscover some of that healing power and wonder.

PART ONE

We have to change our patterns of reacting to experience. For our problems do not lie in what we experience, but in the attitude we have towards it.

Akong Rimpoche

I

············✥············

What is Aromatherapy?

Holistic aromatherapy is a natural therapy and healing art, using essential oils extracted from aromatic botanical sources, to balance and treat the mind, body and spirit. As it is primarily a body contact therapy, aromatherapy powerfully combines the profound physiological effects of massage with the psychological influences of essential oils on the mind and emotions. It must be the most pleasing way to health and good feeling that there is. It smells good, is therapeutically sound and feels wonderful.

Along with the benefits to mind, body and spirit, one of the many aspects of treatment that makes aromatherapy so appealing, is the range of principles involved and the many forms of application and methods of use available. Treatment can be effected by inhalation, baths, compresses and creams, but the most lasting influence is achieved when the oils are applied to the skin by massage. The essential oils are highly concentrated and are diluted before use - cutaneous absorption of the oils through the skin and into circulation takes approximately 30 minutes, not being as instant as initial inhalation, however maximum benefit is achieved when applied to the skin, as the oils remain several hours in the system before they are eliminated via the lungs, skin and urine.

When used with a correct understanding, knowledge and care, aromatherapy can be a viable alternative or complement to orthodox treatment - for countless conditions and for anybody and everybody, as the essential oils treat the whole person, not only the specific symptom. In certain circumstances however, such as when treating cancer patients, massage is not recommended unless under strict medical supervision and specialist guidance. Aromatherapy can be and is used effectively in reducing stress and helping in the care of cancer patients however, in both private and public hospitals, with positive results. (*The International Journal of Aromatherapy* Vol 1 no. 4/Vol 2 no 1 spring 1989.) Due to their high volatility, essential oils can be of particular benefit in hospitals to prevent the spread of infection due to airborne bacteria resistant to antibiotics, antiseptics and disinfectants. Many hospitals are plagued by bacteria resistant to antibiotics, this because of their constant exposure to them in the hospital environment. In 1987, the television programme *Horizon* made a study in a hospital in Melbourne, of patients' reduced response to antibiotics precisely due to this problem. Aromatherapy is regularly used in hospitals in England, and at the John Radcliffe and Churchill hospitals in Oxford, essential oils are being used instead of sedatives and to help both pre and post operative patients recover from the trauma of surgery.

Commonwealth Industrial Gases, part of the BOC group, and a major Australian corporation, is using Bactigas, a mixture of tea tree essential oil and carbon dioxide, as a fine spray misted through the air conditioning system, to benefit "sick buildings" and benefit workers. The anti-fungal and antibacterial properties of tea tree acts against mould, mildew and fungi that thrives in the warm and moist atmosphere of the air conditioning. The programme is also resulting in less respiratory infections, less contamination in food processing areas and a reduction in absenteeism from illness. A company director from CIG notes:

"There has been a marked reduction in absenteeism due to sickness such as colds and flu. Bactigas has helped provide us with a healthier working environment." (IJA vol 3 no 3 - autumn 1991/Tea Tree Oil - Susan Drury, The C W Daniel Co Ltd 1991.)

There are a great many ailments that can be effectively treated with the most natural of all things given to us on this earth, the innocuous weapons Nature has given us in her herbs and plant life. Aromatherapy is particularly effective in helping us to help ourselves, by forms of treatment that cause no stress to our systems, by working in harmony with our own strengths and weaknesses and promoting relaxation and good health. The ever increasing evidence of allergic reaction, adverse side effects and dependency on chemical drugs, is of particular concern during pregnancy and for children. There is no doubt that being pregnant and giving birth can be the ultimate high experience, and the most fulfilling, but it can also be the original "low", and one of the most demanding experiences a woman can face. There could be countless times when treatment is needed to help cope with certain ailments, discomfort and the inevitable tiredness that pregnancy can bring, and at this time more than any other, it is crucial to maintain optimum health and happiness in a safe, non-toxic and non-habit forming way. Being pregnant and knowing the miracle of your child growing within you, is perhaps the most precious time in a woman's life, certainly the time when good health and well being is of prime importance. We are all ultimately responsible for our own health, and during pregnancy and parenthood, for another's too. The care you give cannot be more important than at the very beginning of life, when you and your unborn baby share a common need for good health.

"Aromatherapy", "Essential Oil Therapy", "Osmotherapy", "Aromacology" and many others, are just a few of the many terms used today to describe the use of essential oils for therapeutic use, although the healing properties of plants and herbs has been known about for thousands of years and has occupied a very special place in man's life. The use of herbs and plants is the oldest method of healing disease and pain, and the many myths, medicinal and magical properties surrounding plant life have been recorded in the oldest writings of history.

More than 5000 years ago, records on Egyptian papyrus showed the use and application of aromatic substances, when there was little distinction between perfume, medicine and religious ritual. In those times, a common product had different actions and purpose, in contrast to today, when chemical drugs tend to have specific action. After the infused oils used in ancient Egypt, came the distilled essential oils used in Persia in the 10th century. There is no record of essential oils and distillation before this, although a terracotta still was discovered in Pakistan, carbon dated to be over 5000 years old - so who knows?

René Gattefossé, a French chemist and researcher into the use of essential oils for skin conditions and medicinal use, first coined the phrase aromatherapy. He published his book, *Aromatherapie*, on the subject in 1928, after which a great deal of interest was kindled in essential oils and their medicinal benefits, particularly in France and Italy. Professor Paolo Rovesti, director of the *Instituto Derivati Vegetali* in Milan, continued this research into the influences of essential oils to relieve anxiety and depression, but it was Dr Jean Valnet, a French doctor and army surgeon who contributed most to the scientific validity of aromatherapy. He used essential oils extensively to treat burns and wounds during the second world war, and his book, *The Practice of Aromatherapy* is essential reading.

The Austrian biochemist Marguerite Maury was inspired by a book, *Les Grandes Possibilités par les Matières Odoriferantes*, given to her by a Dr Chabene, who later taught Professor Gattefossé. After moving to France, Mme Mauray spent the major part of her life researching and demonstrating the effects of essential oils on the nervous system, their rejuvenating properties and their influences on holistic well being. She also developed the theory of individual prescription and the holistic approach to the therapy. She was a great force, if not the only one, in establishing the reputation of the therapy in France since Dr Valnet and the second world war. In Britain, alternative therapies were still treated with suspicion. Marguerite Maury was totally dedicated to her work and gained recognition for this devotion by being awarded two international prizes in 1962 and 1967 for her ceaseless research and work in cosmetology and essential oils. In 1968, she died of a stroke aged 73. She worked until she died, her last manuscript at her bedside. Danièle Ryman, a former pupil of Mme Maury, continues her work after more than 20 years, and played a major role in her most wonderful and special book, *The Secret of Life and Youth,* being republished in English by The C W Daniel Co Ltd. Mme Maury still inspires through her words and through her energy. The same company has now republished Gattefossé's famous book.

Robert Tisserand wrote the first general introduction in English on aromatherapy in 1977, another book difficult to write under the pressures of family life and babies! Both he and his book *The Art of Aromatherapy* were responsible for opening the door and introducing one of the most fascinating and neglected therapies to countless English speaking people - at a time when interest in natural therapies was fast developing. He set up the first UK essential oil business in 1974, selling oils directly to the general public, since which time demand has grown beyond all expectation. He and I set up the Tisserand Aromatherapy Institute in 1987, to establish comprehensive and qualified aromatherapy training and to provide a focus for professional interest. This led to the launch of *The International Journal of Aromatherapy* in 1988, to promote awareness of current professional research and to meet public demand.

Many healing properties of plants are fully accepted by leading authorities today, although not so very long ago, when these healing benefits were common knowledge to ancient herbalists, the clash with "authority" would have had them burnt at the stake. Things have improved somewhat today however - but it must be remembered that although herbal and plant therapy has evolved throughout the ages, the majority of medical and scientific attitudes still tend to be in favour of the synthetically produced uniformity of preparations. Some probably still believe in the stake...

There is still a long way to go to unearth the many as yet unknown mysteries of plant life and secrets Nature might share. We are only just beginning to learn of the importance of many therapeutic plants being made extinct by our systematic damage to the environment, as we are also learning about ourselves and our worlds. In 1974 the World Health Organisation made a pronouncement that if the Third World was to achieve adequate health care by the year 2000, then they would have to retrieve their herbal traditions and nurture and develop their traditional systems of medicine, rather than rely on expensive western drugs and chemicals. There is now a "fresh look" being taken at the herbal roots of modern medicine, especially from the once stoically sceptical medical establishments. In France, UK, Germany and USA, a large number of drug companies are marketing phytopharmaceuticals, or plant drug preparations, and there are many papers being published in medical journals on the therapeutic benefits of herbs and plants.

Fortunately, there is now much more scientific and cultural research into aromatherapy and its very many and varied therapeutic benefits. The scientific aspect of aromatherapy cannot and should not be ignored and although research is increasing, the lack of funding prevents the clinical value of the art being "proven" as quickly as it might. Things are indeed changing for the better however, with growing interest in the therapy involving scientists in many disciplines - including biochemists, physicians, biologists, chemists, psychiatrists, sociologists and the perfume industry in particular - all recognising the significance and import of smell and its influence, not least the therapeutic benefits of holistic aromatherapy. With more people in differing professions becoming increasingly aware of the therapeutic benefits of essential oils, this underlines the need for further scientific evidence to establish the therapy as valid, effective and respected. The financial aspect of research always plays a major role, as it does in the profit involved in production.

However, the lack/absence of this laboratory data does not invalidate the success rate of aromatherapy. The countless case studies recording disappearing symptoms, increased immunity, health and vitality along with restoring and promoting the balance between body and mind is abundant evidence that the use of essential oils and aromatherapy is more than valid.

Although many ailments can be effectively treated by the lay person and there are many short courses, weekend seminars and books available on aromatherapy for home use, professional advice from a fully qualified and registered practicioner is always recommended. It should not be forgotten that any diagnosis requires long term medical knowledge, and any doubt about the seriousness of a condition should be confirmed by a specialist. Aromatherapy can effectively complement orthodox and most alternative or complementary disciplines, often combining to great advantage. However, when combining treatments, full consultation with the fellow practicioner is essential in order to gain maximum benefit and response from the patient. If combining aromatherapy with osteopathy for example, the consequent relaxation of the patient can effectively benefit treatment, either before, during or afterwards, particularly with the manipulation so often required in osteopathy. With homoeopathy, if a course of aromatherapy treatment was underway to clear congestion of the lymph system and boost immunity, then a homoeopathic remedy to assist in clearing this congestion would be appropriate, or vice versa.

The majority of us are lucky enough to live in a society where we currently have freedom of choice, and the merits of both orthodox and complementary have their place. Whatever principle, and whether for or against whichever camp, the great progress made in the last century alone to protect us from illness and disease has undoubtedly saved the lives of many. We smile now at the writings of centuries ago, just as we will undoubtedly make our descendants chuckle in the next century (if not before!), but knowledge is a relative thing and there should always be caution against over confidence and pride in what knowledge we currently possess, to the exclusion of an open mind. There is much to learn, and still a long way to go to unearth the many as yet unknown mysteries of "pure" essential oils and holistic aromatherapy, including the many secrets Nature holds for our benefit.

II

-----------◆-----------

How Does Aromatherapy work?

Aromatherapy has a *psycho-therapeutic* action. With or without the countless therapeutic benefits of applying the essential oils in massage, smelling the oils alone influences the psyche, directly affecting mood and emotion and causing response in our central nervous system and brain.

Although there are many methods of treatment and application, essential oils are most commonly used in massage, where the oils are diluted in a vegetable base and applied directly to the skin. The oils are absorbed through the skin by the oily medium of sebum, they pass into the bloodstream and are carried to all parts of the body via the circulation. The oils can influence our systems for several hours, days or weeks, depending on the general health and condition of the patient, although they take approximately 30 minutes to be fully absorbed into the system before being eliminated via the lungs, skin and urine within a few hours. There is much scientific evidence to show the benefits and effect of touch, also the profound influence odour has upon our mind and emotions. Touch and smell are our "close range" or intimate senses, not necessarily sexual but most certainly sensual, and aromatherapy powerfully combines the therapeutic benefits of both, causing deep response throughout the whole body.

Smell has a direct influence on us through the mind, as it is a particularly emotive sense with a direct link to the brain and central nervous system. Smell stimulates the nerve cells and sends electrical signals through the *olfactory bulb* into the *limbic* system of the brain. These receptor cells line the upper part of the nasal tract and are both nerve and brain cells. They live for a month on average, before being replaced by fresh cells, this behaviour not applying to any other brain cells. The genes involved make hundreds of receptor molecules waiting in these cells, ready to capture any passing odour. It is thought, from the new discovery of these genes, that the smell receptor system may be one of the most sophisticated receptor systems in the body. The limbic system is a complex area of the brain, involved in the expression of instinct, self preservation - including reproduction and the care of offspring - mood expression and memory. The limbic system is also known as the emotional centre of the brain.

It is now known that smell has a profound effect on both long and short term memory and emotions, influencing us even when we are not necessaily aware of the effect. The most significant odours should be the ones Nature has designed for us, secreted by the sebaceous glands, and concentrated in areas such as the armpits, groin and breasts. (Any unpleasant odour comes from contact with bacteria.) This pheromonal effect influences a baby's reaction in identifying mother. The fact that breast fed babies recognise their mother more easily by odour than bottle-fed babies, was established in 1985 by Jennifer Cernoch and Richard Porter of Vanderbilt University in Nashville. (New Scientist, page 45, 25/8/90) This reaction can form a direct association with good or bad events. Almost everybody can remember a situation whereby an odour has recreated an association or recalled a long lost memory - cinnamon toast after sledging and happy families, special scents and special people - "Ahhh, it was when...", or "Yeuuch...!"

Vita Sackville West writes about the particularly haunting and beautiful scent of roses in her *Garden Book*:

> *"Some writers would call it nostalgically scented, meaning everything that burying one's nose into the heart of a rose meant in one's childhood, or in one's adolescence when one first discovered poetry, or the first time one fell in love."*

This influence on memory cannot be shown on a brain scan, because we are all conditioned by experience in different ways, but it is possible to show the changes affected in the brain in response to smell stimulation. The Olfactory Research Group at Warwick University have produced a remarkable video showing the brain's response to an odour, and the equally strong response in the central nervous system immediately an odour is perceived.

Response to odour is particularly heightened during pregnancy, when some odours you cannot get enough of, others being completely abhorent, causing a physiological response such as nausea and actual sickness. This is also so when an odour of a substance to which one is allergic is sensed. The ever increasing evidence of allergic reaction, adverse side effects and dependency on drugs is of particular concern, especially during pregnancy and for children. I have an allergy towards coffee, and I still have to avoid the area near the coffee shop when they are roasting the beans, it makes me badly nauseous - not a good recommendation for the friends who own it. Coffee is a good example of the fact that taste is approximately 80% smell, as is the old restaurant adage of selling "the sizzle not the steak" - the tongue only perceives salt, sweet, sour and bitter, the subtlety of taste being registered by olfaction. When the nose is blocked during a cold for example, caviar might as well be cold rice pudding.

Providing certain safety precautions are observed, children react very well towards aromatherapy, their responses being free from any pre-conceived ideas or expectations. Babies respond particularly favourably towards massage and a loving touch, as does the child in us all. At the West London Hospital, baby massage is being practised with great results, with classes in Islington involving aromatherapy & massage in helping babies with eczema, constipation, irregular sleep patterns and general awareness. Communication begins with the very simplest of things - the touch and odour of our mother when we are first born. As we get older, body contact decreases as communication by action and word takes over, yet stresses and strains of everyday living increase. If these stresses and strains are allowed to continue, an imbalance occurs, immunity decreases and ill health results. This is where aromatherapy comes in. Each individual is unique, with specific and exclusive symptoms and causes of ill health and because aromatherapy and the use of essential oils is phscho-therapeutic, acting on the psyche as well as physically, the therapy is highly versatile in treating all manner of conditions. Aromatherapy can also help to boost immunity by its action on the adrenal glands and nervous system, and as essential oils have antiseptic and antibacterial properties, they act against infection. If used in a spray or diffuser, they act efficiently against airborne bacteria by releasing their molecules into the atmosphere. Aromatherapy is particularly beneficial for common childhood ailments and during pregnancy when the use of antibiotics is not recommended.

Researchers at the University of Warwick's chemistry department believe the key to matching the potency of chemical tranquillisers lies in "nature's own tranquilliser", this being a steroid molecule found in human sweat, named *Osmone 1*, which is chemically similar to components of sandalwood oil and other animal musks. Dr George Dodd and Dr Jenkins are co-directors of Warwick's olfaction research group, and their company, Osmotherapy Limited, based at the university's Science Park (Coventry, CV4 7AL), has manufactured the commercial product called *Relax*, currently available from the company by mail order.

There are three basic forms of aromatherapy - *clinical*, *aesthetic* and *holistic*. Clinical aromatherapy has been practised in France for many years, French GP's prescribing essential oils, usually for internal use, for countless infections and disease. Clinical aromatherapy is only practised by those with a thorough background of medical knowledge and the oils have to be of the highest quality.

Aesthetic aromatherapy is normally used as an adjunct to beauty therapy and relaxation, using basic blends of oils or commercially or previously blended oils to work on a superficial level of influence. This sense of luxury and relaxation is certainly of benefit, although usually administered by those without professional medical training and not involved in treating illness. Training in the use of essential oils is usually of a few days.

Holistic aromatherapy brings the complete healing process together and is practised by professionally trained aromatherapists. This involves an in depth assessment of the individual, to recognise and evaluate subtle weaknesses and physical and emotional symptoms. Treatment is given after a thorough assessment of lifestyle, diet and nutrition, exercise and general physical and emotional circumstances have been considered. For home use, other than general assessment, any specific diagnosis should only be made by a professional.

Holistic aromatherapy combines the two most fundamental and primitve senses of touch and smell in a therapeutically beneficial treatment, the essential oils having profound and far reaching influence. Only when our vital organs, our nervous system and circulatory systems are relaxed and unstressed, can we be at ease in body, mind and spirit. The influence of aromatherapy, on mind and physical function is widely accepted. "Take time to smell the roses" - it makes you feel good as something happens inside. Aromatherapy is a simple practice, it's natural, uncomplicated and works beautifully.

"Everything in life should be made as simple as possible, but not simpler."

Einstein.

III

What are Essential Oils?

Essential oils are derived from aromatic botanical sources. The plant material is harvested and the oil extracted when at the height of oil production. Roses and lavender for example, are always distilled in August when the maximum amount of essential oil is in the plant. Depending on the part of the plant containing the essential oil, the essences are extracted by steam distillation, expression, solvent extraction, maceration or enfleurage, the quality of the oils and extraction varying from country to country. Essential oils come from many parts of the world, often from several different countries, and as they are cultivated under differing conditions, organic or otherwise, the oils you purchase can vary considerably in quality and expense.

The south of France used to be recognised as the centre of the essential oil industry, with acres upon acres of fragrant plants and flowers, however, in recent years the French have moved towards synthetics, as has the perfume industry in general, with far fewer aromatics being as naturally produced as they once were. A number of Third World countries are now successfully cultivating essential oil plants and are beginning to dominate essential oil production. Countries as far afield as South America, Australia, Egypt, Turkey and Bulgaria, African countries including Madagascar and the Commmore Islands, are fast becoming prime suppliers of essential oils. Where peasant farmers still use traditional methods of extraction, huge stills can still be seen at the edge of fields, where it is more practical to harvest and distill delicate flowers that would lose their freshness if transported.

Both peasant and factory methods have their place, factory extraction being far more controlled, although in many cases it is impractical to build factories near to the botanical source.

Aromatherapy is already big business, aromatic sources being cultivated on larger and larger scales to cope with the ever increasing demand for essential oils. There are also many synthetic replicas of the essences available and in use, there inevitably being great debate as to the term "pure" essential oil - from the manufacturers of the "exact chemical copy", to the growers providing the oils from a "purely organic" source. There are many suppliers of essential oils, pure, chemical and blended and many varying degrees of quality. Demand is ever increasing as more and more wish to train in the therapy and more essential oils are being bought off the shelf for home use. As demand increases, so does the necessity for high standards of quality control, clarity of marketing and professional training.

Production and transportation costs, along with the basic economics of supply and demand all affect the price of essential oils. When an oil is more difficult to extract, it is obviously more costly to produce. Jasmine for example, cannot withstand the high temperatures of steam distillation, therefore the lower temperature of solvent extraction is used, resulting in an "absolute", this being far more expensive than an essential oil extracted by standard steam distillation. Jasmine has also proved to hold a higher concentrate of essence if harvested during the night when the highest percentage of essential oil is present in the plant. (Most of us have delighted in the scent of jasmine at night and the memories recalled of particular moonlit nights under the jasmine...? If you haven't - you should!)

Both the absolute and the essential oil can be obtained from the same plant, such as rose absolute and rose otto essential oil. To extract an absolute, the plant is washed in alcohol, (macerated or steeped) for anything up to several weeks, during which time the waxes and terpenes separate. It is then filtered by centrifusion, the separate solid becoming the "concrete", which is then distilled at a lower temperature than by normal steam distillation, to give the absolute, or oil, on top of the solvent. During normal distillation, plants are steamed in stills, the beads of essential oil rise up the still, are cooled as they pass through a funnel from the top of the still and form a film on top of the collected water vapour. These waters are usually discarded as they do not retain the odour of the plant, the exceptions to this being rose and neroli (orange blossom). Most toilet waters contain an average of 10% - 15% aromatic water. Eau de Cologne is generally made from citrus oils, these being far cheaper to extract, usually by expression, the pulp and peel producing the essential oil. Jasmine absolute is contained in many perfumes, although usually the more expensive ones, as it is a costly oil to produce.

Essential oils may be extracted from every part of the plant:

Flowers:
Neroli - Rose - Lavender - Ylang-Ylang - Chamomile - Jasmine (absolute)

Leaves:
Basil - Sage - Rosemary - Thyme - Clary Sage

Fruits:
Bergamot - Grapefruit - Orange - Lemon - Lime

Nuts & Berries:
Juniper - Cypress - Nutmeg - Bitter Almond

Seeds:
Caraway - Celery - Corriander

Grasses:
Lemon Grass - Ginger Grass - Palmarosa

Roots:
Oris - Ginger - Calamus - Vetiver

Wood:
Sandalwood - Cedarwood - Rosewood

Bark:
Cinnamon

Gums:
Frankincense - Essential oil from gum is extracted by cutting the bark on either the trunk or the branches, the gum oozes out and is collected, powdered and distilled in the normal way.

Different essential oils may be obtained by using different parts of the same plant. The oil obtained from the cinnamon leaf and the cinnamon bark are completely different, with differing therapeutic qualities, as are the oils from orange trees - essential oil of *orange* from the fruit, *neroli* from the blossom and *petitgrain* which is now from leaves and twigs. The majority of essences are clear in colour, although always check if you are unsure, as the wonderful blue of German Chamomile (due to its high content of *azulene*), may not seem quite so beautiful if it stains treasured linen!

There are about 200 essential oils commercially extracted and some further 500 not specifically for commercial use. Of these, 200 or so are well known in the practice of aromatherapy today, although more and more are being researched and becoming available. Many are variations of existing oils. The content of essential oil varies within each plant, the average being approximately 1 - 2%, although it can be as little as 0.01% in the case of rose, or as high as 20% in some gums. Essential oils are highly volatile substances and they evaporate at different rates. Eucalyptus oil evaporates very quickly compared to sandalwood for example, therefore in a blend containing both these oils, the initial aroma would be of eucalyptus, with sandalwood dominating afterwards. This evaporation rate can be classified as oils having top/high, middle and base/low notes of aroma, a high note essence such as eucalyptus evaporating within the first half hour or so, middle note within 2 - 3 hours and low between 6 - 12 hours on average.

Every oil has a degree of evaporation to be considered when deciding on a suitable blend, a balance is necessary to incorporate essences with top, middle and base notes, affecting the physical as well as emotional levels. Too many top note oils, such as most citrus oils, would not be long lasting enough, whereas oils with a predominantly base note, such as ylang-ylang, would be too heavy. Like herbal remedies, the oils must be blended to suit individual needs. They are not symptomatic treatments as such, because they have an influence on us both physically and emotionally. Aromatherapy can be used to treat anybody (although not always in massage - see contra-indications) because the oils work on the whole person, not just the ailment or symptom. An understanding of how the oils work and at what levels, along with how they behave together in a blend should be coupled with your own sensitivity and intuition. It should also smell wonderful!

Essential oils are all inflammable and this can clearly be shown by squeezing the peel of an orange into a flame. The oil ignites, so great care should be taken when using burners, or on light bulb rings.

The shelf life of the oils can vary considerably. Generally, the more citrus the oil, the shorter shelf life it has (Lemon, Grapefruit and Orange go off quickly and turn cloudy) and a lot depends of course, on how fresh the oil was when purchased. As quality never comes cheaply, always buy your oils from a specialised source and from a supplier who hopefully has a high turnover, thus ensuring the oils are never in bulk stock for long periods of time and are as fresh as they can be when you buy them. Unfortunately, at the time of writing, suppliers do not as yet date the oils. Heat, light, damp and oxygen, which causes the oils to oxidise, all adverseley affect essential oils. Always keep your oils away from extremes of temperature, and ensure the tops are tightly closed when not in use.

The prices of essential oils can vary greatly too. As a rule, you get what you pay for. Many oils are sold as blends, or diluted in carrier oils, especially the more expensive essences, such as Rose, Jasmine and Neroli. If this is so, it should be clearly shown as a dilution. The undiluted essences you buy should not as a general rule feel oily, as if they do, they have been diluted in a carrier oil and you are not buying the concentrate. There are many "aromas" you can buy, but as we are not concerned with just perfumery, only the natural essence should be used for therapeutic purposes.

Essential oils are fast acting against bacteria, fungi, viruses and micro-organisms and have a broad spectrum of action. They have a selective action in that they can stimulate our natural immune stystem, yet act on isolated bacteria in a safe, non-addictive way and without side effects. Antibiotics undoubtedly have their place, but the disadvantage of taking them is that they also kill off the friendly bacteria in the process. Whenever antibiotics are taken it is common for Thrush to develop, so if you are susceptible, advise your GP (see A - Z). Essential oils are also skin active in that they are readily absorbed into the skin and blood stream, where they can have a particular effect. They are cytophylactic (cell vitalising), although some more so than others, in particular lavender, neroli, bergamot and chamomile. They all have a psycho-therapeutic effect.

Essential oils are extremely subtle, yet highly potent and it is not the case in aromatherapy that if you use more, a greater effect is achieved, this is especially so when the synergistic effect of the oils is considered. Every oil used in a blend should work not only in harmony with the patient, but also be compatible with other oils used. Some oils when used together, produce greater activity than when used separately - never confuse the idea that more is better. The addition of a minute amount of a particular oil to a blend can change its whole influence. Their effects can be as regulators, stimulants, sedatives and euphorics, to help with anything from gall-stones to grief. When you use the oils, think "holistic aromatherapy", as problems in one area are undoubtedly linked to others. Everything is related, negative emotional and mental processes commonly leading to physical disorders. Holistic treatment is concerned with all aspects of well-being, inside and out - and at all levels.

Essential oils are highly concentrated and should not be used directly on the skin by the lay person except for tea tree and lavender and only in specific cases. The carrier oil or base oil with which you create your blends, should not be too aromatic and not interfere with the therapeutic action of the aroma of the essential oils. The oils you use should be vegetable, nut or seed oils as these are readily absorbed into the skin, and should also be cold pressed, thus avoiding any additional chemical processes. The most commonly used base oils are as follows:

Almond:
This is Sweet Almond oil. (Bitter almond oil is toxic - hydrocyanic acid/cyanide!) Sweet almond is inexpensive compared to some oils, is light, almost odourless and ideal for massage.

Avocado:
Avocado oil is heavy and green and contains vitamins A and E. Although the vitamin E content in this oil acts as an antioxidant, helping to preserve the life of your essential oils, the E content is not as high as that of wheatgerm oil. Avocado oil is often used as an alternative to wheatgerm, as those with wheat allergies can sometimes react unfavourably to wheatgerm oil. It is usually used as an addition to base oil due to its heaviness, in a 10% dilution.

Jojoba:
Jojoba oil is a waxy oil that will solidify at cold temperatures. It penetrates the skin well and comes from a bean which grows in the arid deserts of North America. It is used as a replacement of whale oil. Jojoba is well known for its beneficial uses on the skin and was widely used by Indians for its varied benefits. Like Avocado oil, Jojoba can be used in addition to the base oil in a 10% dilution.

Peach Kernel:
Peach Kernel is a very light oil and the ideal carrier oil for facial massage.

Wheatgerm Oil:
Wheatgerm oil is high in vitamin E and other proteins, minerals and vitamins. It helps to prevent oxidisation of the essential oils. Use a 10% dilution with another base oil. CAUTION:

Those with a wheat allergy may have a sensitivity to wheat-germ oil. Take a skin patch test 24 hours before intended use, to test for reaction.

Other base oils include: Apricot Kernel, Corn oil, Evening Primrose (10% dilution), Grapeseed, Hazelnut, Olive (10% dilution), Peanut, Safflower, Sesame Oil (10% dilution), Soya Bean and Sunflower oil.

Although the actions of some essential oils can be "categorised" to a degree, they all have certain similarities. They are all antiseptic, antibiotic, cytophylactic, fast acting and psycho-active, the differences being that some are more beneficial than others in a particular instance. Lavender and tea tree for example, are both excellent in skin complaints, both healing, both antiseptic - but for burns, lavender is second to none and for its highly antiseptic and anti-fungal properties, there is nothing to beat the actions of tea tree. Essences enhance each other to improve the overall effect, but as a general guide, some oils can be classed into five groups.

Regulators:

Bergamot	Frankincense
Geranium	Rose Absolute
Rosewood	Chamomile

Stimulants:

Eucalyptus	Juniper
Peppermint	Rosemary
Tea-Tree	Basil

Sedatives:

Lavender	Marjoram
Chamomile	Orange Blossom
Sandalwood	

Euphorics:

Clary Sage	Jasmine
Rose Otto	Ylang Ylang
Grapefruit	

Aphrodisiac:

Jasmine	Ylang Ylang
Patchouli	Clary Sage

IV

······· ✦ ·······

Methods of Use

Although there are many forms of application and methods of use, an aromatherapy treatment has the most lasting influence when applied through massage, as it is several hours before the oils are eliminated from the system via the lungs, skin and urine. Direct inhalation of the oils also has an effect, although the influence is not as long lasting as when applied via the skin. During massage, both have an effect, the lungs directly absorbing properties of the essences, but most are absorbed through the hair follicles of the skin, the sebum being the oily medium through which the essential oils are absorbed into the bloodstream and circulated around the system.

During pregnancy, more than any other, it is essential to maintain good health and consciously develop relaxation and times of rest. Essential oils can be used in all manner of ways to enhance that feeling of calm and peacefulness, both inside and out, for you and your baby. Massage, aromatic baths, meditation, breathing exercises, rest and relaxation all help to create a peaceful and harmonious environment for you both. During pregnancy or not, when the body's immunity and "cope-ability" factor is low, a weakness in this imbalance shows itself through ill health. The use of essential oils in aromatherapy goes far beyond mere application of "this oil for that problem", as in the many and varied methods of use, essential oils and the holisitic approach to the art of aromatherapy can effectively return the body from an imbalanced state to one of harmony and well being.

To create a unique harmony with maximum therapeutic effect needs thorough knowledge of the oils, their many subtle yet powerful uses and also a degree of knowledge of the many and varied systems of the human body. It needs to smell pretty good too. The intuitive side of the therapy also plays a high profile, especially so in choosing the suitable synergistic blend of oils for maximum benefit to treat the relevant condition. Increased potency does not necessarily increase with dosage. A synergistic blend of two or more essential oils is chemically different to the sum of the combined separate essential oil properties, and in the right proportions, is unique and powerful in its own right. Never confuse the idea that more is better.

A diagnosis should be avoided, unless absolutely sure of the condition, as accurate diagnosis requires long term medical knowledge and should be left to the specialists; however the use of applied kiniesiology, and reflexology can also play an important part in an aromatherapy treatment in helping to establish a more specific treatment and relevant oil or oils.

The methods of use below give the recommended quantities of pure, undiluted essential oils and are to be used as a guideline. Where a specific blend is necessary, refer to the relevant entry in the A-Z section. Essential oils are highly potent and highly concentrated and where less than one drop of oil is required, such as in blends for babies or young children, use a glass pipette available from most chemists. Keep a separate pipette for each oil.

Massage:

For use in massage, essential oils are blended with a vegetable carrier oil or base oil. The usual blend of essential oil to carrier oil is 2 - 3%, however a good guide is to measure one drop of essential oil to 2mls of carrier oil. This gives an average $2\frac{1}{2}$% dilution.

For an approximate guide to blending and quantities, use the following:

20 drops	= 1ml of essential oil
5ml	= 1 teaspoon
10ml	= 1 desertspoon
15ml	= 1 tablespoon

For example - $2\frac{1}{2}$% dilution:

	mls:	%:
Essential Oil..........	$1\frac{1}{4}$ (25 drops)	$2\frac{1}{2}$
Carrier Oil	$48\frac{3}{4}$	$97\frac{1}{2}$
	50ml Bottle	100%

i.e.   10 drops in 20ml of carrier oil
        25 drops in 50ml
        50 drops in 100ml etc.

Empty bottles can be bought from your chemist and once carrier oil and essential oils are mixed, the blend will last for 2 to 3 months. Don't forget to date and keep a note of the blend for future use. Any remaining oil can be used in the bath to "top up" any treatment.

Compress:

The compress may be either cold or warm, again depending on the treatment. A piece of absorbent material such as a cotton hankerchief, a sterilised flannel or cotton wool may be used. To the cooled, previously boiled water, or chamomile/ peppermint tea, add the relevant oil or oils in the specified amount, "swish" the oils over the surface of the water (they do not mix well in water), and using the material, soak the oils off the surface of the water. Apply to the area in need for at least 10 minutes. For stomach or back pain where a warm compress is required, a hot water bottle placed on top of the compress will give additional relief. For a cold compress use a medical freezer pack, crushed ice, or for speed, a bag of frozen vegetables, peas being the best, as they mold to the area well.

Air Freshener:

All essential oils are anti-bacterial, some more than others. For use as an air freshener, use your favourite aroma by placing a few drops on the radiator, on the carpet, in the hoover bag whilst hoovering, or on a light bulb ring especially for the use of essential oils. Do take care to only use colourless oils if using on linen or furnishings that will stain. In addition to the effect on air borne bacteria, don't forget their use as mood enhancers.

Inhalation:

To a bowl of hot water, add the relevant essences, usually 2 or 3 drops, place a towel over your head and to cover the bowl, then lean over and inhale the vapours. Keep your eyes closed, as the vapours can be quite strong, and breathe deeply through your nose .

One or two drops of a suitable oil can be put on a handkerchief or tissue and sniffed when required. This is instantly effective and particularly inobtrusive if you need help with your driving test, exams, dentist, shopping with baby or life generally!

Internal Use:

Although essential oils are used by the food, medical and cosmetic industries, they should not be taken internally except under the strict guidance of a fully trained practitioner. Some oils are highly toxic and although not on sale to the general public they are available. A list of the hazardous oils is given under toxicity, along with a section on contra-indications.

Gargle:

For a gargle, use Tea Tree and add 2 to 3 drops of the essence to a glass of water, mix thoroughly and gargle away.

Douche:

For the treatment of vaginal disorders, see a professional therapist.

Bath:

Run the bath to the temperature required - too hot can be debilitating - and close the bathroom door and windows. Add the essences to the bath making sure that the oils are mixed thoroughly in the water and to prevent any neat concentrates of oils coming in contact with delicate skin when you sit down... Soak it all away for as long as you can, usually a minimum of 10 minutes, and breathe deeply. Spoil yourself completely and take the 'phone off the hook, turn the lights off, light a candle and relax to your favorite music. Any number of oils can be used, but as a general rule no more than a combination of four and maximum of 10 drops to a full size bath.

Diffusers/Vaporisation:
There are many types of diffusers available, all especially made for use with essential oils. The oils are heated and the vapours are released into the atmosphere. Essential oils are inflammable and the materials used in diffusers should be of a non-flammable material. These are usually made of clay, metal or glass and the oils are heated by electricity or by candle flame. Take great care when using a light bulb ring, not to get oil onto the bulb as this can drip onto the attachment or ignite.

For a home made vaporiser, add 6 - 10 drops of your chosen oil or oils to a large bowl of very hot water. If used in a young child's or baby's room, make sure they are unable to reach the bowl and follow the appropriate guidelines for the maximum amount of drops.

Ointments/Creams:
These can be made by adding essential oils to vaseline, coconut oil, beeswax and vegetable oil or aqueous cream, all of which are available from a good chemist.

For 30mls:

7g unrefined Beeswax (just under 7mls)

23ml veg oil

20/21 drops of essential oil(s)

Place shredded beeswax and oil in a pyrex bowl inside a pan of water over a gentle heat. Stir until the wax has melted into the oil, maximum temperature should be 40° - 45°C. Place the bowl into a pan of cold water to cool and as it begins to thicken and solidify once more, add the essential oils, mix well and pour into containers. This makes a more solid cream which liquidises when in contact with the warmth of the skin. *Lavender, Bergamot and Tea Tree, in equal proportions, makes a good antiseptic cream.*

The same method applies if not using beeswax. Gently heat the oils, stirring together until blended. If required, add rose or orange flower water, half the quantity of the vegetable oil, adding the water very slowly and in tiny amounts whilst stirring or beating briskly. This can be done in a blender on a very low setting. Stir in the oil(s) when the cream is well blended and cooled.

Both vaseline and aqueous cream are bland and can also be used for ease of preparation. Add the oils in a 3% dilution to the cream, again unless otherwise recommended, and if vaseline is in a tube, one drop of oil per inch of cream. Mix well together in the palm of your hand and apply.

Don't forget to label and date your creams.

V

············ ✦ ············

Contra-Indications
Toxicity & Dosage

The remedies given are for home use, using the most commonly used essential oils. Always seek professional advice from a fully qualified aromatherapist in cases where more specialist information is necessary, and if in any doubt whatsoever about symptoms, check with a medical practitioner.

Do not treat anyone with cancer, heart disease or any other potentially fatal condition, unless under the strict guidance of a fully qualified aromatherapist who must have medical clearance and be in full co-operation with the patient's doctor or specialist.

Never use essential oils neat on the skin, apart from Lavender and Tea Tree, and then only when specifically directed.

Never use aromatherapy or massage when the patient has a migraine and never in the eyes.

Never massage directly over any skin infection, inflamed bites or stings, varicose veins, recent fractures or scar tissue, bruises, acute inflammation, or if the patient has a fever temperature.

The therapeutic benefits of an aromatherapy treatment are without doubt, however reactions to treatment can vary considerably. In order for an imbalance to be corrected, a change has to occur to stabilise any disharmony within the system. Sometimes the patient will feel worse before feeling better, then as treatments are increased or changed to remain in balance with the condition, will begin to improve. Others will feel a positive change after or even during the first treatment, and some will have swings between both. If there is a steady improvement which begins to tail off, the blend needs to be changed to compensate for the difference in condition.

Dosage:

Unless otherwise stated for specific conditions in the A - Z section of the book, follow the guidelines below. When more, or less than the average amount of essential oil is recommended, use a glass pipette, available from most chemists, which gives approximately one quarter of a drop from a standard bottle of essential oil. Avoid using the same pipette for different oils.

When the number of drops to use in a blend is also given in brackets, this applies to an alternative method of application.

Newborn:

Avoid using essential oils to treat newborn babies until they are at least one week old, then only Lavender or Roman Chamomile and maximum 1 drop of each, well diluted to a maximum of a quarter of the standard amounts given.

From 3 months to 18 months:

Use a quarter of the standard amounts given.

From 18 months to 7 years:

Use half the amounts given.

From 7 years to 14 years:

Use from half to the maximum of 2 - 3 % of the amounts given (i.e. maximum 15 drops in 30mls, 25 drops in 50mls, etc.).

TOXICITY LIST OF ESSENTIAL OILS

The following oils should not be used.

Aniseed
Bay (Pimenta racemosa)

Birch Tar
Bitter Almond (Hydrocyanic acid)
Boldo Leaf
Calamus
Caraway
Cassia
Cinnamon Bark
Clove Bud
Clove Leaf
Clove Stem
Cormint
Costus
Elecampane
Fennel (Bitter)
Hyssop
Lavender-Cotton
Savory
Mugwort
Mustard
Ocotea cymbarum
Origanum
Pennyroyal
Pine Pumilio
Rue
Sassafras
Sage
Savin
Savory
Southernwood
Tansy
Tarragon
Thuja
Thyme
Wintergreen
Wormseed
Wormwood

During pregnancy do not use the following oils unless specifically directed, or under the strict guidance of a fully qualified, professional aromatherapist:

Basil	Lemongrass
Clary Sage	Marjoram
Cedarwood	Myrrh
Cypress	Parsley
Fennel	Peppermint
Jasmine	Rose
Juniper	Rosemary

Avoid Chamomile, Lavender, Geranium and Melissa in the first three months of pregnancy unless specifically directed.

A properly trained and qualified aromatherapist, will know the contra-indications to massage and the use of certain essential oils in certain conditions, however skin sensitisation or allergic reaction is a different thing altogether. If there is any doubt at all about possible allergic reaction, do a skin patch test 24 hours before use, to test for any sensitivity and possible reaction. Fortunately it is rare for there to be any adverse reaction to unadulterated essential oils, however not all oils are "pure". If any reaction is experienced, it is normally when the oils have already been blended, such as with the addition of wheatgerm oil for example, or with a synthetic addition, or when there is an allergy to some perfumed toiletries. If bought from a supplier registered with E.O.T.A., (The Essential Oil Trade Association), there is some guarantee that the oils will be unadulterated, as the association is a professional body that regulates essential oil standards – to suppliers, the public and to the food and flavour trade. The oils sold by retailers registered with the E.O.T.A. have to be checked – initially, and at random times subsequently, to ensure continued quality, so always purchase your oils from a registered supplier.

VI

······ ❖ ······

Pregnancy

"Making Babies" will mean a whole new language of emotion for you and your partner. It will also mean learning a new language of words and terms, some from you, when you try to understand and explain how you really feel, but most will be new medical terms. If you ever have any doubts, or feel at all confused by what you hear or read, always ask your doctor or midwife to explain. In the A - Z section of this book, you will find some of the more common terms explained.

As far as when your baby was conceived, you and your partner may know exactly when this was and could even feel "different" from that moment onwards. Those first feelings taking place deep within you are very unique and very special. In the weeks that follow, your awareness will increase as your body changes to cope with the needs of the tiny life growing within you. During pregnancy, your body will change faster than it has at any other time - for some it is a shock and they feel hideous and fat, for others fascinated by the changes, they will feel wonderful and beautiful (if not quite all the time...) Whatever your feelings, be honest with yourself, if you feel awful, and many women do feel extremely rough, especially during the first three months coping with all the vast hormonal changes going on, then take it easy - it's a learning *and* growing time!

If your periods are of average length, you will actually be about two to three weeks pregnant when you miss your first period. In medical terms however, your pregnancy is dated from the first day of your last menstrual period (LMP) so you may not know you are expecting a baby until you are "officially" around five to six weeks pregnant.

An average pregnancy is classed as being of forty weeks duration and is divided into three terms known as trimesters. The pleasures and concerns of pregnancy alongside the emotional and physical changes, often fall in with each trimester. Every woman is different and every pregnancy is different, and for many women, 40 weeks can seem a very long time, for others it can pass all too quickly. It takes this time to build up the relationship between mother and baby - and 40 weeks is not a long time for you to prepare and adjust to the fact that you will be a parent for the rest of your life. By the time you actually get to meet each other face to face, even though you and your baby have both "been through it", the long build up is more than worth it - you actually get to meet! The reality of your soon to be role as parent, will gradually increase as the presence of your child growing within you becomes more evident. From the very first union of sperm and egg, you and your baby have a life long relationship, whether you feel happy, excited and "blooming", or thoroughly ill from the first moment of conception, those weeks will absorb all the totally miraculous happenings going on within you, and give you time to get to know your baby, and yourself. Apart from all the physical and emotional changes you have to absorb, your baby also has to have time to change from a single cell to a highly complex organism with millions of cells.

When you first guess that you might be pregnant and a missed period confirms your thoughts, then a pregnancy test is advisable to be totally sure. The sooner you know you have a baby growing within you, the sooner you can consciously avoid all risks not only to you, but to your unborn child. The risks of dangers to the baby are greatest during the first trimester when the baby's organs are forming. Many drugs can cross the placenta to your baby and cause possible abnormalities in the foetus. Even drugs taken without thought for common ailments such as headaches, nausea or sleeplessness can be harmful, especially at the beginning, so the sooner you know, the sooner you can tune in to your intuition and start using aromatherapy.

The various hormones produced by the endocrine glands (in women, including the ovaries and placenta) are responsible for the many changes a woman will experience during her life as her body matures, from menstruation to menopause. These hormones are responsible for the increased physical and emotional changes occurring during pregnancy and birth - especially *oestrogen* and *progesterone*, levels of which dramatically increase during pregnancy and which play a major role in adapting the body to the countless needs of pregnancy and birth; *prolactin*, essential for ovulation and breast feeding; *relaxin* produced by the placenta to soften tissues and ligaments in the body in preparation for birth; *adrenalin, noradrenalin* and *endorphins*, also part of the autonomic nervous system, and which have a major influence on mood and emotions - and pain! Optimum hormonal balance is the aim to maintain health and well being and to avoid severe emotional swings. Certain essential oils have an influence on these hormonal mood swings, and some such as Clary Sage* and Geranium* can also stimulate or normalise certain hormonal secretions. The oils are delicate, subtle, yet can have a profound effect on the physical and the psyche.

Every month on average, a ripe egg, or ovum, is stimulated by hormones produced by the anterior pituitary gland and released from one of the ovaries to travel down the fallopian tube to the uterus. The ovaries secrete the hormones oestrogen and progesterone and although mainly secreted by the ovaries, small amounts are also produced by the adrenal cortex, the placenta (and the testes in the male). Progesterone prepares the breasts and uterus for gestation and is only present in the circulation after ovulation, oestrogen is secreted throughout the menstrual cycle and controls female sexual development. Both natural and synthetic oestrogen is used in the treatment of menopausal disorders, to inhibit lactation and in oral contraception. Both oestrogen and progesterone are responsible for preparing the lining of the womb (or uterus) for pregnancy. This lining becomes thicker and engorged with blood ready to receive and nourish the embryo

* See contra-indications

if fertilisation occurs. Once pregnancy begins, progesterone continues to be secreted as it also prevents the further release of eggs from the ovaries.

If fertilisation does not take place, the secretion of oestrogen and progesterone gradually ceases, the thickened lining of the uterus is shed and menstruation occurs, all under the control of hormones and the hypothalmus. The levels of these hormones, previously hundreds of times higher than in a non pregnant woman, drop dramatically within minutes after birth and by the second or third day, the levels are very low, therefore assisting the body to return as quickly as possible to its non pregnant state. It is common at this time for the "post natal blues" to occur and now is the time to make use of all the valuable oils that had to be avoided during pregnancy.

Most of the common problems of pregnancy are not serious and can be considerably eased by natural therapies. Refer to the appropriate entry in the A - Z section of the book, however if anything occurs that you are not happy or unsure about, seek professional advice immediately. Do try to make every antenatal appointment, as any queries you may have can be answered, and regular checks on you and your baby can be made. Contact your GP or midwife if you experience any of the following:

Excessive headaches, dizziness or vomiting.

Sudden or pronounced swelling of feet, ankles, fingers or face.

Increased white or discoloured vaginal discharge.

Any vaginal bleeding.

Abdominal cramps.

Any fall or accident.

FIRST TRIMESTER

WEEKS 1–4: In most cases, ovulation occurs approximately fourteen days before menstruation, whatever length of cycle you have. Each egg lives for an average of 24 hours after release from the ovary, so intercourse has to occur within these 24 hours for fertilization to take place. During ejaculation, some 3 to 4 million spermatozoa are released into the vagina. Each has a head carrying the genetic material and a long tail enabling it to move in the fluid medium. The mucus in the cervix is thinner at this time, making it easier for the sperm to travel. Most leak out but some swim up the cervix into the uterus, into the fallopian tube, are attracted to the ovum and stick to its surface. Only one sperm will penetrate the egg, except in the case of multiple birth, and fertilisation occurs when the genetic material of both mix. The egg then loses its attraction and the other sperms drop off. From this vital moment, the first cell of your baby is born.

The fertilized ovum is then propelled along the fallopian tube, dividing quickly from a single cell to a small mass of cells until it finally reaches the uterus after about 4 days. This mass of cells, looking rather like a blackberry at this time, is formed of two layers, the outer becoming the placenta, the inner one your baby.

The sex of your child is determined by two of the 46 chromosomes - 23 from the mother and 23 from the father. When these 46 unite, all the characteristics of your baby will have been determined for life. Some abnormalities at birth or that appear in later life are caused by chromosomal abnormalities. An example of such is Downs Syndrome. Certain diagnosis can be made by examining cells, either before pregnancy or at an early stage in gestation. (See *amniocentesis, weeks 15–18*) Genetic counselling for couples with a history of hereditary disease in families is available, however many congenital abnormalities are caused by viral infection and the effects of drugs taken by the mother at the early stage of pregnancy. Before the twelfth week, the placenta which acts as a barrier to protect the growing baby is not fully developed.

At about one week after conception (week 3 after LMP), implantation in the uterus occurs and tiny *villi* from the cluster of cells penetrate the uterine blood vessels to reach your bloodstream, where they begin to be nourished. Your maternal blood is carrying all the vital nutrients for your baby, this vital connection maturing to form the placenta, which will help her to survive until birth.

By the end of the first month and at the end of this miraculous journey, the cluster of cells is now implanted in the uterine wall, and begins life as a tiny embryo. At this time you might well feel different, with tender breasts, certain dislikes and even nausea and heightened emotional response. You will more than likely feel particularly tired for no obvious reason and might already suspect that you are pregnant.

WEEKS 5–8: By the beginning of the second month, a pregnancy test would show the presence of the hormone *HCG*, (*human chorionic gonadotrophin*) in your urine and blood. This hormone is produced by the placental cells. Placental hormones are also now beginning to influence your digestive system, possibly leading to nausea and constipation. (See the relevant entry in the A - Z section). A reduction in appetite may lead to lack of energy and increased nausea, so remember to try and eat well and maintain regular bowel movements.

Your baby at this stage already has the beginnings of a nervous system, spine and brain, the heart is beginning to beat and rudimentary eyes, ears, mouth and limb buds are appearing. By the end of the second month, she is still only about an inch long, but her bones are beginning to harden and all her major organs are in place although not yet developed.

WEEKS 9–14: During these weeks, if not before, you will begin to notice tight clothes and your waist will probably be vanishing. At this time, breasts and nipples can begin to feel extremely sensitive. Both hair and nails will be growing more rapidly than usual, hair often changing for the better or sometimes worse, as with your skin. This will settle down once hormonal levels become more established, but in the meantime, make sure you eat well, take as much fresh air as you can and rest as often as possible. Make sure you look after your teeth too, as during pregnancy, gums become spongier and more prone to infection. Make an appointment at the dentist - dental treatment is free for pregnant ladies.

By week 10, the embryonic period has ended, and your baby's human characteristics are now clear, her kidneys are even beginning to produce urine. At 12 weeks your baby is approximately 5.5 cms/$2\frac{1}{2}$" long, from head to bottom, and weighs less than 20 gm/1oz. During weeks 11 - 14, as the nervous system matures, movements become more activated and coordinated, swallowing and breathing reflexes are now present and the movements of lips and head turning are part of the sucking reflex. The placenta now covers one area of the uterus, which has now emerged from the pelvic cavity and may be felt above the pubic bone and any initial feelings of nausea and possible vomiting should begin to diminish.

SECOND TRIMESTER

WEEKS 15–18: Although some food preferences may still remain, you will probably now begin to feel a lot better. The second trimester and middle stage of pregnancy is the most enjoyable, as you have become accustomed to being pregnant, and much tiredness has disappeared. You might even feel creative and energetic! If you want a holiday, now is the time to go, whilst you feel secure in your pregnancy but not too large to be uncomfortable.

Baby is now growing very quickly, her heart is beating strongly and the breathing reflex is well established as she inhales and exhales amniotic fluid. She is also rehearsing functions of digestion and elimination by swallowing the fluid and passing it through her bladder. She now has tiny finger-nails and movements are more coordinated - she can suck her thumb and make facial expressions. At 16 weeks, baby is about 10 cms/4" long, and weighs 120 gm/$4\frac{1}{2}$ oz.

During the second trimester, you may have an *ultrasound scan* done. The test for *amniocentesis* can only be done during the second trimester, between 16 - 18 weeks of pregnancy, this is done to detect possible abnormalities in the foetus if such a risk is present. A sample of amniotic fluid is drawn out by a needle and tested, results of which are available after approximately 4 weeks. This can be an extremely stressful time, so do use the essential oils to help if applicable.

Begin gentle exercise now, especially pelvic floor exercises.

WEEKS 19–22: Around this time if not before, you will begin to feel the first definite movements of your baby, normally just when you are still, relaxed and wanting to go to sleep! Hearing is now well established, and any loud noise could make her jump. She could begin to enjoy music from now on, and don't forget to talk to her. Her skin is now covered in *lanugo*, a fine downy hair, and *vernix*, a white, cheesy substance that protects baby's skin in the watery environment of the womb. This is sometimes present at birth, but will soon go. At week 20, baby measures about 15cm/6" and weights 300 gm/11oz.

Towards the end of this month your increased weight might result in the discomforts of back pain, cramps or varicose veins, so be well aware of correct posture, and rest as much as you can with your feet above your heart.

WEEKS 23–26: Baby's cycle of rest and sleep is now established, with reflex movements being well demonstrated. You might even feel hiccups. A baby born after week 26 may well survive, although she will not be mature enough to survive without help. At week 24, baby measures around 20 cms/8" and weights 640 gm/1lb 5 oz.

The increased pressure from your enlarged uterus on your bladder will cause the need for frequent urination, and your increased weight also making night time sleeping more disturbed, so do rest as much as you can at this time.

Third Trimester
❖

WEEKS 27–40: During month seven, the membranes covering your baby's eyes part, and her eyes open for the first time. The colour of her eyes is not usually fully developed until a few months after birth, until that time nearly all babies eyes are blue.

At week 28, baby is thought capable of sustaining life out-side the protection of your womb. She now measures around 23 cm/9", and weighs about 1 kg/2lb 2 oz. Although not fully mature, with modern special care facilities she has a good chance of survival. At week 32, baby measures about 26.5 cm/10½" and now weighs around 1kg 700/3lb 12oz. In the eighth month, the endocrine systems in both you and your baby are actively preparing for birth, both physically and emotionally. Baby will respond to your moods and emotions through your hormones passing to her through the placenta. Pressure from the uterus which now almost fills the abdominal cavity can make breathing difficult. Also practice contractions (*Braxton Hicks*), can be quite strong, the uterus noticeably hardening and relaxing. This pressure can often cause heartburn, rib pain and discomfort in the pelvic region until the pressure is released any time now, when baby's head engages in the pelvis and pressure is released. Bliss - and you are on your way! Antenatal visits are weekly now, and the antenatal classes are getting quite serious. By now you will be already learning about labour and how to "pant, pant , pant," (instead of 'puff, puff, puff'!).

During the ninth month, baby's consciousness is well established, with progressive organisation of brain activity. The placenta stops growing but continues to function, and baby could be born at any time, so be ready. Make sure you have your oils already blended and labeled, both for you and your partner, case packed if going to hospital and baby's room and layette ready. At week 40, baby's approximate length is 37 cm/14½" and weighs about 3 kg 250/7lb 1oz. (All lengths and weights are average, and are taken from crown to rump as this is a more accurate reading from a scan). Head to toe measurement is, on average, around 50cm/20½".

By now your ligaments and joints will have softened in preparation for birth. You will probably begin to feel centred and more meditative. You might feel the reverse however, and the "nesting" instinct may take over, with you tidying, cleaning and working harder than you have in months. I recommend the former! Baby has now probably quietened down and is moving much less and you are probably becoming quite nervous, impatient, excited or relieved, - pregnancy has become a familiar state after all this time...

No matter how many times you have gone through the stages of birth in your head, each labour is highly individual, so no matter what you have decided, be flexible for your sake, your partner's and your baby's. It is bound to be a completely different experience to the one you planned or hoped for, sometimes better, sometimes worse. Don't forget to make use of the essential oils. They can and will help tremendously, both physically and emotionally.

Birth is classed in three stages. Your labour may start when the mucus plug sealing the cervix is dislodged. This is known as the *show*, and may be tinged with blood. You may feel contractions (which can be felt as lower abdominal ache or lower backache), or breaking of the waters (which may be felt as a slow, warm trickle or a gush). Ring your midwife or the hospital if you are in any doubt, as labour can begin with any or all three of the above.

The first stage of birth is when your uterus begins to regularly contract, and continues until the closed cervix ripens and opens up. The end of the first stage is when you are said to be "fully dilated", usually about 10 cms and wide enough for baby's head to pass through.

The second stage of labour is usually much shorter than the first and is when you must stay as relaxed as you can. Contractions change in nature, becoming more expulsive, longer and more frequent, helping baby down through the birth canal and into your arms.

The third stage is when baby is born and you finally get to meet each other. The placenta then separates from the lining of the uterus and is expelled by further contractions (not normally noticed!). Your baby and family are now born.

There are many reasons why labour may have to be started by induction, either for your safety or your baby's – but whatever happens, don't forget to be flexible, as no two births are ever the same and it would be a miracle in itself if labour and birth went exactly according to plan!

Also see Birth, Babymoon & Bonding in the A–Z section.

PART TWO

··· ✥ ···

Scent, of course, is not only biologically the oldest but also the most evocative of all our senses. It goes deeper than conscious thought or organised memory and has a will of its own which human imagination is compelled to obey.

Laurens Van Der Post

VII

Essential Oils

Arnica:

There is an essential oil from Arnica, however it is highly toxic and should never be used.

Homeopathic Arnica however, is invaluable for its use in the treatment of bruises and sprains, or shock - either for internal use or as a cream.

Basil - Ocimum basilicum:

Basil oil is marginally toxic and should not be used during pregnancy or on children. It is a general stimulant oil and could be an irritant to those with sensitive skin if used in too strong dosage. However, it is an especially useful oil, hence its inclusion here - ideal for giving a degree of "alertness" if one is lacking in sleep or function. It is an uplifting oil, ideal for use after pregnancy, for partners or anyone else.

All lovers of good food are familiar with the gastronomical delights of fresh basil. Basil has a longer history than most aromatic herbs, coming from its native India to Europe via the Middle East. The Egyptians passed their knowledge on, and Pliny and Dioscorides recorded basil in their works in the first century AD. There are more than 100 varieties of basil, its wide range of uses including seasoning, herbalism, aromatherapy and its association with magical and religious rites. It has a long history of use in Indian traditional medicine and according to the Brahman religion, it was held as a sacred plant, bringing spiritual and physical protection to the wearer. The name is derived from the Greek *basilicon*, meaning a royal remedy.

The essential oil is taken from the leaves of the plant. It is cultivated in France, USA, Egypt, Madagascar and the Seychelles, is pale yellow in colour and the odour is spicey, slightly peppery, fresh and green, with a strong top and middle note of aroma.

Basil has more influence on the mind than emotions. It is a refreshing and restorative oil and a good brain stimulant. It helps with confusion, apathy, depression, poor memory and general mental fatigue and as it is also an antispasmodic oil, basil can help in strengthening the nervous system and releasing tightness in bronchial and digestive problems. Basil is a general tonic, can relieve nervous tension, flatulence and nausea and aids digestion. Dr Valnet recommends the use of basil oil for scanty menstrual periods and for whooping cough.

In medieval Europe, basil was credited with the power of relieving the pain of a woman in labour, if she held a root of basil and a swallows feather in her hand... speakers in the Fang tribes of Africa chew basil leaves to give them inspiration and assurance.

Benzoin - Styrax benzoin:
The Benzoin tree is cultivated in Thailand, Java and Sumatra, the absolute coming from the gum of the tree. Benzoin is one of the classic ingredients of incense along with frankincense and myrrh and was burnt in ancient times to drive away evil spirits. Compound tincture of benzoin is also known as *Friar's Balsam* and is recommended for inhalations. It is reddish brown in colour and is warming, drying, comforting and rich in odour. It blends well with most oils.

The warming benefits of benzoin are particularly helpful in all "cold" conditions, such as influenza, colds, coughs and bronchitis and for the relief of gout and rheumatoid arthritis. Its comforting warmth is also beneficial in times of sadness or loneliness and it combines well with neroli or rose in these cases. Robert Tisserand recommends its use in treating "cold affections of the genito-urinary system, and may be used in cystitis, albuminuria, or any conditions where there is infection or discharge, such as spermatorrhoea, gonorrhoea, and perhaps leucorrhoea."

Madame Maury says of benzoin: "This essence creates a kind of euphoria; it interposes a padded zone between us and events." Because of its warming properties both internally and externally, benzoin can also have a positive, calming, yet euphoric effect.

Bergamot - Citrus bergamia:

Bergamot fruit is from a tree, the oil being extracted from the rind. It is farmed primarily in Italy where it was originally cultivated. Bergamot oil is yellow/green in colour and the odour is rich, citrus and sweet. It has a strong top and middle note of aroma and blends well with most oils. Compared to most other citrus oils, bergamot has a warmer, more superior odour and is widely used in the perfume industry. Because of its refreshing, yet relaxing qualities, it is a classic ingredient of Eau de Cologne.

The aroma of bergamot oil makes most people smile, is known to uplift and inspire and can be used effectively in cases of anxiety, stress or depression. It is particularly effective against skin infection and disease and as with most citrus oils, is notably antiseptic. Bergamot is a very versatile essential oil, blending well with most oils and being pleasing to both males and females, not being too sweet. Dr Valnet recommends Bergamot for loss of appetite, colic and intestinal infection.

Although Bergamot is of special use in skin treatments, it is phototoxic in that it can cause a skin reaction when exposed to UV light, from either a sunlamp or from sunlight. This can cause blemishes or uneven tanning, so do not use it if you expect to be out in the sunshine. This can also apply to Eau de Cologne and some commercially produced perfumes and toiletries containing bergamot oil. (Earl Grey tea has bergamot added to it, giving it its scented flavour. There is however, no problem in "taking tea" in the sunshine.... enjoy!)

Black Pepper - Piper nigrum:

Pepper was probably the earliest spice known to man, and was a highly prized luxury. It came originally from the

Malabar coast of India, and became of such value that it was used to pay taxes and levies in place of coins. As demand soared, the Portuguese explorer Vasco de Gama opened up the sea route to India and the spice islands, since which wars over the pepper trade have been hot and fiery.

Essential oil of black pepper is extracted from the berries or peppercorns of the plant. It is cultivated in Java, Sumatra, Malabar and Penang and is normally amber in colour, although this can vary depending on the age of the oil. As you would expect, the odour is hot, biting and strong, so only a small amount is ever needed.

Black Pepper is a stimulating oil, its principle areas of action being on the respiratory, digestive and urinary systems. It blends well with the fortifying benefits of frankincense and sandalwood and can restore tonus to lax, smooth muscles. Black pepper is an effective rubefacient (local stimulation of skin), and with diet and exercise can help to eliminate cellulite. It gives relief from stiff muscles and with its pronounced stimulating action on the digestive tract, can help with constipation, flatulence, loss of appetite and with atonic dyspepsia.

The warming benefits of black pepper are good for colds, influenza and fever. Externally it is good for warming general aches and pains, can give relief for rheumatoid arthritis and can ease any physical or emotional "coldness", apprehension, lethargy or melancholy. In any sluggish condition, black pepper can stimulate, however be aware of the distinction between stimulating and irritating and follow the rule of less is more. Increased potency does not necessarily increase with dosage. A synergistic blend of two or more essential oils is chemically different to any of the oils used separately and in the right proportions is unique and powerful in its own right. Never confuse the idea that more is better. Patricia Davis in her excellent book, *Aromatherapy an A-Z*, recommends the use of black pepper for dancers and athletes for use before training or performance, to prevent pain and stiffness, so bear this in mind when you start jogging again after baby is born!

Cedarwood - Cedrus atlantica:

Cedarwood oil is marginally toxic in high concentrations and should not be used during pregnancy.

Juniperus virginiana is known as Red Cedar and is grown in North America. It is closely related to the Yellow Cedar from which*Thuja* essential oil is obtained. Thuja is highly toxic and should never be used in aromatherapy.

The oil from Cedrus atlantica, or Atlas Cedar, is frequently used in aromatherapy and is cultivated in Morocco. The name comes from the the Semitic root word signifying "power" or "strength", a suitable description of this stately tree. The wood contains a high concentration of oil and is very aromatic. There are few trees left from the great forests of Lebanon Cedar used by the ancients for their palaces and temples, including Solomon's great temple in Jerusalem, and latterly, because of the great demand for cedarwood furniture.

The Egyptians used cedarwood oil in the mummification process, also as an ingredient for cosmetics, for ships, furniture and coffins - a somewhat varied medley of uses. It is still used today in traditional Tibetan medicine. The oil is clear in colour and its aroma is similar to sandalwood, being warm, woody and masculine. The aroma is rich at all levels, is long lasting and thus good as a fixative as it blends well with most oils.

As with sandalwood oil, cedarwood can have a pronounced effect on mucus membranes and is good for use in pulmonary conditions as an inhalant for all catarrhal conditions, coughs and bronchitis. The therapeutic properties of cedarwood have long been recognised, including its benefits for skin conditions, acne, oily skin and dandruff. It is popular with males as it has a more "masculine" aroma than most oils. It is also excellent as an insect repellant. Judith Jackson states that it encourages sexual response - try it!

Chamomile (German) - Matricaria chamomilla/
Chamomile (Roman) - Anthemis nobilis:

There are several types of Chamomile, two of which are commonly used in Aromatherapy, German and Roman. The

German tends to grow wild and is known as the True or Wild Chamomile, the Roman is nearly always cultivated. The name *Matricaria,* from *matrix* (womb), gives a clue to the use of this herb by the ancients. Dioscorides and Galen prescribed it for female disorders and fever and chamomile tea is still an aid to relieving female conditions and easing childbirth.

German chamomile is an annual herb, the oil being extracted from the flowers and seeds of the plant. It is cultivated in England, Hungary, Germany and Belgium. It is a wonderful deep blue in colour, this due to its high azulene content, is sweet, mellow and hay-like in aroma and has a strong odour at all levels.

Roman Chamomile is a perennial herb commonly grown as a scented lawn, in England there being a famous chamomile lawn at Buckingham Palace. The essential oil is extracted from the flowers of the plant. Roman chamomile is pale blue or pale yellow in colour and is more fruity in aroma than German Chamomile, the strength of aroma not being as strong.

The anti-inflammatory properties of either chamomile are without doubt, especially in dermal inflammation, and although their use is more physical than emotional, chamomile is soothing and calming, often helping to break the vicious circle of tension and effect. Its uses include treatment for nervous upsets, feverish conditions, menstrual and menopausal pain, dull aches and pains, including cramps, rheumatic and gout pains, skin eruptions, acne and scabbing, dermaitis, eczema and psoriasis.

Roman Chamomile, like German, is very calmative and has positive benefit for many women's complaints such as menstrual pains, premenstrual tension, heavy or prolonged bleeding and menapausal dificulties. It is also good for colic and teething problems.

In chamomile's homeopathic application, camomilla grains can be placed in baby's mouth to help with teething pain. It has long been valued for its use in lightening fair hair and is widely used in modern shampoos. Never use any essential oil in or near the eyes, however chamomile has been noted for its use in treating eye conditions such as conjunctivitis, and a cold tea bag placed over the eyes can bring effective relief.

Either Chamomile is excellent to use in treating children, as it is especially mild yet therapeutically sound - although Roman has a lower note of aroma than German. Its calmative properties are ideal for use as a mild nerve sedative for children, as a febrifuge, and especially for teething problems. Chamomile is a particularly healing oil in that it stimulates white cell production and reduces inflammation. Azulene is a principal constituent in Chamomile, and to quote Dr Valnet:

"Azulene is a fatty substance discovered in the essence of Matricaria (camazulene). It possesses healing and antiphlogistic properties which have been studied chiefly by the Germans, and in France by Caujolle. Numerous experiments have shown its remarkable effectiveness in treating various inflammations of the skin, eczema, leg ulcers, vulvar pruritis, urticaria, and also chronic gastritis, colitis, cystitis and certain kinds of asthma.

"The bacteriostatic effect of azulene is produced at a concentration of one part in 2,000 against Staphlococcus aureus, haemolytic Streptococcus and Proteus vulgaris in particular. Infected wounds have been healed using concentrations of from one part in 85,000 to one part in 170,000."

Clary Sage - Salvia sclarea:

Clary Sage is sometimes known as "Clear Eye" from the Latin word *Clarus* meaning clear. In the Middle Ages it was used for eye complaints. Clary Sage is a small biennial herb, the essential oil being extracted from the flowering tops of the plant. The plants are cultivated in Spain, USSR and France. The oil is pale yellow in colour or clear, and the odour is nutty, floral, and slightly sweet. It has a strong middle and base note and blends well with other oils as it lasts well. It is commonly used as a fixative in perfumes.

Clary Sage is a subtle yet powerfully effective oil and is most valuable for use in stress-related conditions. It is a good anti-depressant, giving a sense of well-being. It has been likened to the effect of a good bottle of champagne, although I must add that it does not have this affect on everybody...

Because of this sometimes effect, it is not recommended that the patient drives anywhere after a treatment. It is also a gentle sedative and quietens the nervous system, is effective against states of anxiety, stress and nervous disorders and can help with high blood pressure. It can be a most effective euphoric and has been likened to an aphrodisiac, being effective in cases of mental and sexual debility. It is particularly beneficial in helping with post natal depression, premenstrual tension and period problems. Avoid using Clary Sage during pregnancy.

Cypress - Cupressus sempervirens:

Doctor Leclerc recommended other members of the medical profession to prescribe Cypress under its Latin name, this to prevent patients being put off by the gloomy association of Cypress with cemeteries. Cypress trees are evergreens, and sempervirens, meaning ever-living, is probably the reason why they are in abundance around cemeteries, especially in Mediterranean countries.

The oil of the Cypress tree is extracted from the leaves and fruits and is cultivated in the Mediterranean. The oil is clear or pale yellow in colour and is refreshing, woody and spicey with a hint of pine. It has a strong top and middle note of aroma.

Cypress is known for its anti-spasmodic and vaso-constrictive properties and is one of the most astringent of essential oils. It is effective for oily skin, menopausal conditions, circulatory maladies, including those of the venous system (varicose veins, and haemhorroids) and incontinence. It can help in drying up colds, with influenza, coughs, whooping cough, fever and excess perspiration. Dr Valnet mentions it for its benefits in drying up excess foot perspiration, Hippocrates and the Assyrians for uterine conditions and haemorrhoids, and Galen for diarrhoea. In addition to being a deodorant, Cypress is also an insect repellant and has been most valuable on the animals in our houshold - for their benefit and ours. It acts well on the female reproductive system, and is of value in menstrual disorders. Avoid using Cypress during pregnancy.

Eucalyptus - Eucalyptus globulus:

There are many varieties of Eucalyptus, the above being the most favoured for essential oil production. Eucalyptus is grown in Australia, Tasmania, China, Spain, California and Brazil. The oil is extracted from the leaves of the tree and is clear in colour. The odour is fresh and powerful with a very strong aroma at all levels, so only a little is ever needed in a blend.

Eucalyptus contains a powerfully antiseptic essential oil and is good for any pulmonary problems. It is an effective room freshener, ensures a healthy atmosphere and makes an ideal inhalation in helping with colds, influenza, sinusitis, sore throats, coughs and bronchitis. Dr Valnet mentions its use for asthma and pneumonia. It is an effective decongestant and expectorant and is also good for cuts and wounds. It has been known as the "fever tree" due to its capacity to soak up water, and it was normally planted in marshy regions, ideal breeding grounds for infection and fever. It is an effective insect repellant, especially when used with Bergamot, and although often planted near houses, it does however poison the ground of the surrounding area, preventing other plants from growing.

Eucalyptus with high levels of eucalyptol are used for medicinal purposes, whilst others are used in perfumery. Eucalyptus globus contains a high percentage of eucalyptol (80-85%). Dr Jean Valnet gives specific information on its bactericidal properties - "used in a spray, an emulsion of 2% essence of eucalyptus kills 70% of ambient Staphlococci" (*The Practice of Aromatherapy*, page 122). More serious infections due to staphlococci include pneumonia, bacteraemia (bacteria in the blood), inflammation of bone marrow and enterocolitis (inflammation of the colon and small intestine).

Used in its natural state, eucalyptus oil has more effect than eucalyptol in isolation, which is extracted and used pharmaceutically in pastilles and as a vapour to relieve catarrh. As Patricia Davis says in her book, this illustrates "once again the fact that essential oils in their natural state are often far more effective than the single chemical constituents so beloved of chemists."

The antiseptic and healing properties of this oil are well known and the psychological angle of "if it smells or tastes strong and potent, then it must be doing some good..." is certainly worth remembering when mixing blends including eucalyptus oil.

Evening Primrose oil:

Evening Primrose oil comes from a plant related to the willow herb family. It is not widely used in Aromatherapy however it is of particular value, hence its inclusion. EPO, normally available in capsule form, is invaluable for its pronounced influence on countless conditions commonly helped by Aromatherapy, particularly in relation to female conditions. It is promoted for the relief of many conditions, including atopic eczema, mastalagia (breast pain - both cyclical and non-cyclical), PMS, multiple sclerosis, rheumatoid arthritis and asthma. Although a remarkably safe treatment, patients with a history of epilepsy should avoid EPO.

There is much on-going research into the benefits of Evening Primrose oil, the market being worth over £35m and expanding. EPO is rich in essential fatty acids and contains high levels of *gamma-linolenic acid* (9% GLA), when compared with most other edible oils - along with *cis linoleic acid*, known to be essential for human health. GLA converts in the body to form prostaglandins, which act as vital cell regulators and are highly reactive, but short-lived. GLA is also found in breast milk. New sources of GLA are being sought and these include borage/startflower oil containing 18% GLA, and javanicus and mould oil containing 16%. (The Pharmaceutical Journal: June 1991)

Evening Primrose oil is of great help to countless sufferers of PMS, in regulating heavy or scanty periods and balancing hormone irregularity. Women suffering from PMS are believed to be low in essential fatty acids and prostaglandins, this leading to an excess of prolactin and the resulting mood changes so often associated with this condition. (Nursing Times - April 1991: Bernadine Say, Midwife, University College Maternity Hospital, London)

In a study on the effectiveness of Evening Primrose oil made by *Here's Health* magazine:

"*Stomach cramps and bloated stomach disappeared*"

"*Period pain reduced from severe to absent*"

"*Premenstrual symptoms greatly reduced in first month and almost disappeared second*"

"*Dramatic effect, no monthly row with husband*"

Fennel - Foeniculum vulgare:

Fennel was well known to the ancients and was used by the Romans, Greeks and Egyptians in their dishes. It was a principal ingredient of sack, a popular drink in Shakespearian times and Dr Culpepper recommends its use as an antidote for poisonous herbs and mushrooms.

It is commercially grown in Europe. The essential oil being extracted from the seeds, is clear in colour, with a distinctive odour similar to aniseed. Because of this strong odour and its marginal toxicity, it does not mix well in blends, should only be used in a very weak dilution and not at all during pregnancy.

Fennel has been shown to have an oestrogenic action, which indicates its use in menstrual and menopausal problems, also its use in increasing milk production in nursing mothers. It has been known to effect the female reproductive system, probably due to the hormone in its structure being a form of oestrogen. It was interesting to note that one of the smells that neither I nor my friend could stand even a whiff of whilst pregnant or breastfeeding, was fennel - either the oil, the toothpaste or the herb in the garden, and neither of us had any problem during pregnancy or with lack of milk. It has been shown to me time after time that the odour of the oil that you prefer, is the one that you tend to need, and vice versa. It is quite pointless in making a blend which is not pleasing, with no influence on the health or happiness of the patient.

Fennel is good for all digestive disorders, including colic, flatulence, indigestion and nausea. It is both spasmodic and antispasmodic as it is classed as an adaptogen essential oil. This means it has a normalising effect in instigating a reaction to rectify imbalance. Its action on regulating the action of the intestines and on peristaltic movements being an aid to the relief of constipation and flatulence. The decongestant benefits of fennel have been suggested for aiding weight loss, this probably due to its diuretic action in aiding the problems associated with fluid retention, however any form of diuretic should not be used without supervision, as misuse can lead to kidney problems.

Fennel oil can be used as a substitute for peppermint oil as Peppermint is not to everybody's taste. The oestrogenic action of Fennel is because of the high content of anethol (50 - 60%), a plant hormone similar to oestrogen. Hippocrates and Dioscorides recommended its help for wet nurses to aid the secretion of milk, Diosocrides also recommended its use as a diuretic for those who can only urinate "drop by drop". Fennel spice is often added to babies gripe water and drinks, and it is often an added ingredient to toothpaste and mouthwashes as it is good for mouth infections.

Frankincense - Boswellia thurifera:
The tree from which frankincense oil is extracted, is cultivated in Somalia, China, Ethiopia and Southern Arabia. The oil comes from the gum, is clear to pale yellow in colour and is fresh, green and woody with a hint of pine, this due to its pinene content. It has a strong middle and low note and has a dry, fortifying scent with little sweetness. It works well in most blends.

Frankincense has the effect of slowing down and deepening breathing, the ensuing meditative calm bearing on prayer. As with myrrh and benzoin, frankincense has been burnt for ceremony and ritual use for thousands of years.

Frankincense is a rejuvenating oil, is comforting, soothing and fortifying. It is effective on fearful people and particularly those in need of a cuddle, either spiritually or otherwise. It can help with respiratory infections and asthma, and is effective for conditions of the genito-urinary tract. The fortifying action of frankincense gives tonus to loose skin and can help with engorged breasts. Its comforting actions on the emotions give strengh to those who dwell in the past, or who suffer anxiety or hurt from past events. It can be a most useful oil for use during pregnancy.

Garlic - Allium sativum:

Garlic has been known as a shield against illness and has held high rank in the realms of magic, medicine and religion in most lands throughout history. It is a well known panacea.

Belief in the magical power of garlic extended to Sweden where the cattle had cloves hung around their necks to protect them from the Trolls. However, science confirms the many medicinal uses of garlic, mainly due to it being a formidable antiseptic and germicide. Garlic has been recorded inhibiting the growth of cancer, toning up lymph and curing glandular disorders. The workers on the Pyramids were given a daily clove of garlic to prevent maladies.

There is of course an essential oil of garlic, and it is without question the most pungent and repulsive of smells and is strong enough to clear a room in five seconds flat. It has its uses of course, as it is one of the most powerful of all antiseptic oils, but as the smell is so unpleasant, unless you are a masochist, it is generally (widely and wisely) avoided in aromatherapy. The benefits of garlic are without any doubt, there being much specific literature and many statistics to prove the point, but as an essential oil for use in aromatherapy, particularly for use during pregnancy and for children and the family, it is to be avoided. However...Hippocrates suggests "a clove of garlic, clean it, remove the skin and insert as pessary, and the following morning discover whether the woman's breath smells of garlic, if it does, she will conceive; if not, she will not." (The choice is entirely yours...!)

The Spanish say that if everybody ate garlic, there would clearly be, "absolutely no problem..."

Geranium - Pelargonium graveolens and odoratissimum:

We are all familiar with pelargoniums, commonly known as geraniums, and their such joyful contribution to any garden or windowbox - although perhaps not so much the profoundly harmonising effects of the essential oil. Geranium is cultivated in Réunion, France, North Africa, Egypt, China, and USSR. It has a fresh, very green, slightly rosy scent, with a strong top and middle note of odour. It mixes very well with most oils.

Geranium was held in high esteem by the ancients, to heal wounds, cuts and sores and mend fractures. It has many applications, however the special property of geranium oil is of its harmonising properties and its effect in balancing emotional extremes. It is a very cleansing oil and can help to regulate nervous tension and hormone imbalances, especially during menstruation and menopause. It is also effective in adding tone to the skin and treating some skin conditions due to the astringent and antiseptic properties of the oil - although its use should be avoided in cases of dermatitis, as exagerrated reaction has been recorded.

Geranium has an affinity with the adrenal cortex, which governs the secretion of both male and female hormones by other organs and its actions are on any conditions where there is a hormone imbalance or fluctuation. For home use, Geranium should be avoided during the first trimester of pregnancy, and only used in low dilution for the remaining time, unless under the guidance of a professional aromatherapist.

It is a very useful oil to regulate physical, mental and emotional imbalances and because of its subtle yet powerful neutrality, should not be underestimated. Valnet recommends the use of Geranium for engorged or congested breasts, sterility, swelling of the legs and lumbar pain.

Grapefruit - Citrus paradisi:
The oil of the grapefruit is extracted from the rind of the fruit. It is cultivated in Israel and the USA and is pale yellow in colour. It has a fresh, sharp, bitter-sweet odour which is strong at all levels.

Grapefruit oil is refreshing and uplifting in its benefits, with a specific action on the gall bladder, liver and kidneys. (The limonene in the oil has been shown to break down small stones.) It is cleansing, can aid digestion and act as a tonic. Grapefruit can also aid in drug withdrawal with its actions on eliminating toxins. Its actions are similar to those of lemon oil.

Jasmine - Jasminum officinale and grandiflorum:
Jessamine is the old English name for Jasmine. It is grown as a bush and the absolute is gained from the flowers. As it takes

such a vast quantity of jasmine flowers to make the essence, it is expensive - however, as with rose oil, only a very little is needed as it is so strong. You should get what you pay for when purchasing jasmine, a cheap alternative is not the thing to buy for therapeutic use.

Jasmine is cultivated in Morocco, Egypt, Algeria and France and is dark yellow/orange in colour. The odour is deep, warm and thick, floral and heady, and is strong at all levels. It is an ideal oil to mix in a blend and works particularly well with citrus oils as it is so long lasting.

Jasmine is used primarily for emotional and stress related problems. It is euphoric and aphrodisiac and an excellent anti-depressant, being so warm, full and positive. Because of its actions on the uterus, jasmine is invaluable during childbirth. It can strengthen contractions, yet relieve pain and due to its anti-depressant quality, can help with post natal depression.

Throughout history, jasmine has been reputed to be an aphrodisiac. It acts well upon the emotions and relieves tensions and fears, usually the seat of impotence and frigidity. Jasmine has great influence on both male and female, its mellow and warming actions on the emotional levels are parallel with its physical benefits of relaxing and rounding out tenseness and rigidity. It can have a remarkably powerful effect on some, so be sure of your own mood when you use it on your partner!

Juniper - Juniperus communis:

The essential oil of juniper comes from the berries of the juniper bush which is a member of the pine family. The plant is cultivated in Italy and Yugoslavia and is clear in colour. The odour is balsamic and woody with a hint of pine, the strength of odour being weak.

Juniper is known to have many and varied uses and has a special use in urinary tract problems. The berries contain numerous beneficial substances such as organic acids, resins and tannins and it has a high terpene content as with citrus oils. Juniper can promote the excretion of uric acids and excess toxins and is of help with cystitis, kidney stones, gout and rheumatoid arthritis. It is also recommended to help with sciatica, lumbago and cramps. It is a powerful diuretic and antiseptic and can eliminate bacteria involved in urinary infection, also helping to increase urine flow and so expel toxins. In homeopathy, under the name of *sabina juniperus*, it is prescribed in cases of threatened miscarriage and metrorrhagia, (bleeding from the uterus other than menstruation), however avoid the use of juniper essential oil during pregnancy, this primarily due to its action on the kidneys.

It was burnt in the hospitals of Paris during the smallpox epidemic of 1870, and was burnt in public places during epidemics of plague and cholera. Hippocrates used juniper to protect Athens against one of these epidemics, the juniper being burnt in houses, streets and squares.

Since Biblical days, juniper has been considered a magic plant and has often featured in legendary tales and holy stories. The oil has also been effective in relieving water retention and easing painful menstruation.

Lavender - Lavandula angustifolia and officinalis:
Lavender has been used for thousands of years to disinfect, as a carminative, sedative, a tonic and to heal, the Romans using it in their bath water. Lavender is a herb, the essential oil being taken from the flowering tops of the plant. It is cultivated in France and Tasmania and the oil is clear or pale yellow in colour. The odour of Lavender is sweet, floral and slightly woody and has a good middle strength of odour, making it ideal in any blend.

Lavender has many and varied benefits, is a general tonic and fortifying on the body, and gently sedative on the mind and emotions. As it is a cytophylactic and stimulates cell renewal, it is particularly beneficial in skin diseases, ulcers, sores and wounds. It is extremely and speedily effective against burns and a bottle should always be kept within easy reach in every kitchen. It can neutralise stings and bites (bees, wasps, mosquitoes and nettle stings), help to reduce pain and prevent infection. It is an especially valuable oil in that it is calming, quietening, yet gently strengthening.

Lavender is effective in releasing tension so often associated with painful or scanty periods. Just a short sniff can calm troubled nerves and depressed spirits.

Constant reference throughout history is made to the healing properties of Lavender, including Saint Hildegarde, the Benedictine abbess famous for her visions and her learning who wrote about the virtues of Lavender. It is a restorative oil with countless pleasing properties and is safe and subtle in its influence on mind, body and spirits. Lavender oil will also keep linen fragrant and deter moths.

Lemon - Citrus limonum:

Lemon oil is very similar to essential oil of grapefruit. It is extracted from the rind of the fruit and is mainly cultivated in California for commercial use. It is clear to pale yellow or green in colour and is sharp and fresh, being strong at all levels.

Lemon oil is antiseptic and anti-bacterial and has a wide range of uses, from oily skin to influenza. It is medically recognised as an antiseptic and can be used as a hypotensive for arteriosclerosis. Even a few drops can kill the bacillus of cholera, diptheria and typhoid. Lemon juice rids oysters of 92% of their bacteria, in addition to being delicious with any shellfish. Its common culinary use, particularly with fish, has undoubtedly prevented many "dodgy stomachs". The English Navy was the first to issue lemons to crew at sea for more than 15 days, to prevent scurvy.

Lemon oil has a high limonene content, and helps to dissolve stones in the kidney or gall bladder. It is highly effective against infection, both internal and external, with its ability to stimulate the body's own defence mechanisms. It is a good astringent and expectorant and is particularly effective for respiratory problems and oily skins. It has a tonic action on the lymphatic system and can help rid accumulation of toxins in the body. Dr Valnet also recommends its use for anaemia, brittle nails and capillary fragility (varicose veins and nosebleeds). Lemon oil also has an effect on clearing skin blemishes and improving skin tone. Like most citrus oils, lemon is a good insect repellant.

Lemongrass - Cymbopogon citratus:

Lemongrass as its name implies, is a type of grass grown in China, Madagascar, Guatemala, India, West Indies and the U.S.A. It is a herb and is commonly used in oriental cooking. Lemongrass has a strong odour at all levels and evaporates steadily. It has an oily, fresh, citrus aroma and is yellowy brown in colour.

Lemongrass is a powerful antiseptic and bactericide and is known for its use in treating infection and fevers. It is an effective nerve tonic and works well in helping stress related weaknesses and improving muscle tone. It is strengthening as opposed to stimulating and for any muscular aches or lactic acid build up, it combines well with rosemary oil. As lemongrass has a similar smell to verbena, or lemon verbena, the two oils are often confused. They are two completely different plants, the oil from verbena (*lippia citriodora*), being extracted from the low oil producing flowering stalks of the plant and is thus more expensive. The oil from lemongrass is extracted from the finely chopped grass stalks.

Lemongrass, as with most sharp, lemon scented essential oils, can be an effective room freshner and deodoriser and can also help repel insects. It has been used at the Radcliffe infirmary in Oxford, along with Tea-Tree, Geranium and Lavender to replace chemical disinfectants and antiseptics.

The main chemical constituent of lemongrass oil is citral, which if isolated or made synthetically and used on the skin, can cause skin irritation. However, lemongrass oil in its natural state does not cause the same reaction. In tests, it was shown that the other constituents of the oil safeguard the toxic effects of the citral content in the oil.

The effectiveness of lemongrass in stimulating stress-related weaknesses has been shown to help in encouraging milk production and digestion.

Marjoram - Origanum marjorana:

Of the types of marjoram, origanum marjorana, or sweet marjoram, was known by the Greeks as "joy of the mountains". Marjoram is a herb and the Romans knew it as a symbol of peace and happiness. The oil is extracted from the leaves of the plant, the odour is spicy and warm, the strength of aroma being weak. It is cultivated in Europe, Egypt, Hungary and Poland and is pale yellow in colour.

Marjoram is a powerful sedative, an anaphrodisiac (the *opposite* of aphrodisiac, just to be clear!) and can lower blood pressure. It is therefore not recommended for use in depression, for those with low blood pressure, or during pregnancy. It can act effectively in helping with grief and hyper-anxiety states. Dioscorides says it combats acidity and flatulence, whilst Aristotle reports that a tortoise having eaten a snake will immediately eat marjoram to prevent death. Don't try it.

The warming, relaxing action of marjoram works effectively to soothe tired, tense muscles and can relieve the pain of rheumatism and arthritis. It is particularly beneficial in releasing any stress related conditions, such as menstrual or intestinal cramps. The warming, sedative properties of marjoram eases any respiratory difficulties and relaxes both mind and body. Its effect in lessening response, both physically and emotionally can be beneficial in the short term, but as with all oils, prolonged use should be avoided. All blends should be regularly changed in aromatherapy, to pace the variety of changes within and the reactions to treatment. Apparently, a common remedy for singers to protect their vocal cords and preserve their voices, is to use an infusion of marjoram sweetened with honey. It depends on how often you sing lullabies I suppose!

Melissa - Melissa officinalis:
Melissa is a perennial herb native to southern europe and Asia. It has a delicate, uplifting and refreshing aroma, is clear to pale yellow in colour and blends well with most oils.

The therapeutic benefits of Melissa have been recorded by many, in particular its positive effects on the over sensitive, melancholic or those who suffer from nervous disorders or anxiety states. It is a tonic rather than a stimulant, and is effective as a digestive, stomachic and carminative oil. Melissa can promote relaxation and good sleep and as it is a very gentle oil, is safe to use over a long period of time or with delicate or frail people.

As with chamomile, melissa is soothing both physically and emotionally, and because of its gentle, soothing and restful benefits, is useful in cases of shock or distress. Allergic rections can be effectively treated with melissa, as can asthma and respiratory difficulties. It has a cooling, calming effect in cases of fever and asthma, with an antispasmodic action on the bronchi. As it eases tension and stress, melissa oil is of particular use in regularising painful or irregular periods. Its relaxing properties are gentle yet effective, as a general tonic on the mind and the emotions, with an affinity for easing tension often being the cause of problems during menstruation, the menopause and female infertility.

Myrrh - Commiphora myrrha:

The Myrrh bush grows in north Africa and Asia in very dry conditions, the oil being extracted from the gum. The essential oil is a rich, reddish brown and the odour is musty, ancient and curative. As with frankincense, myrrh was widely used in ancient times in perfumes, for incense and in medicines. It is not the sweetest of aromas, can be sticky when too cold and is not suitable for baths as it does not mix well.

Myrrh should be used in small quantity due to its marginal toxicity level, and should not be used at all during pregnancy, this due to its use as an emmenagogue to promote menstruation.

However, Myrrh has been shown to be effective in treating mouth problems, such as ulcers and piorhoea (rotting gums), hence its inclusion here. It is the ingredient of some toothpastes today. Myrrh was also used in Egyptian times to preserve bodies in the mummifying process, and although will not make wrinkles disappear, the "preserving" benefits of myrrh were used in cosmetics, facial masks and other concoctions. It is of benefit to dry or chapped skin, and as with frankincense, is beneficial in bronchial congestion and infection, colds and sore throats.

Myrrh is antiseptic, anti-inflammatory and healing. It was also the principal ingredient in *megaleion*, a perfume used in ancient Greece, and it was carried for use on battle wounds to promote healing. It is an effective oil to use in cases of wasting or weakening.

Myrrh has been used for therapeutic benefits for thousands of years, been recorded in many writings and has stood the test of time. It is effective on slow healing wounds or spots, especially where the skin is moist. (According to Classical myth, the mother of Adonis was changed into myrrh...)

Neroli – Citrus aurantium (amara)/Citrus vulgaris and bulgaradia:

Neroli, from the flowers of the bitter orange tree, is produced in France and Tunisia and is thick yellow in colour. The odour is richly floral, refreshing and revivifing and it has a strong top and middle note of aroma.

Neroli is a very special oil. It has profound influence on nervous conditions such as palpitations or any stress related problems. It is calming, comforting and quietening, being particularly beneficial in situations of shock or distress. It can be effective against nervous diarrhoea, indigestion and insomnia and has been known to help with broken veins, stretch marks and scarring.

The orange is a symbol of innocence and fertility, although Atlanta might not have thought so... She was the swiftest of all living mortals, and would only marry someone who could beat her in a foot race. She would kill the losers so there was never a second best. Aphrodite, the godess of love, decided to help a nice, respectable sort of chap called Milanion, as she felt sorry for him, so she gave him some oranges. At the beginning of the race, he dropped one after another and Atlanta was entranced, not having seen anything like an orange before, so Milanion won the race. They got married, and Atlanta settled down at long last, to become a housewife and mother - the symbol of innocence and fertility...

For many, myself included, neroli oil in a blend is one of the most beautiful of all oils, being invaluable in any cases of vulnerability, grief or "littleness". Although it can have very positive influences on the emotions, neroli is also particularly valuable in skin care. It is a gentle and comforting sedative, is a great comforter in times of anxiety or stress, is an antidepressant and also has aphrodisiac properties.

Neroli can effectively relieve nervous tension and is a useful oil to use against insomnia. For the height of luxury and utter bliss, neroli combined with jasmine and/or rose is a very special experience and the *créme de la créme* of an aromatherapy treatment.

Orange - Citrus aurantium (amara and dulcis)/Citrus vulgaris and bigaradia:

Essential oil of orange is extracted from the peel of the fruit by simple pressure, from the fruit of both the bitter and sweet orange tree. The odour is typically citrus, with a strong odour at high and middle levels.

The properties of oil of orange overlap with those of neroli, being antidepressant, mildly sedative and having a normalising and anti-spasmodic action on the effects of anxiety or stress. Oil of orange is not as subtle as Neroli can be, as it is a more cheerful oil and slightly more refreshing. If neroli proves too expensive, then orange oil is a good substitute.

Parsley - Petroselinum sativum:

Parsley essential oil should not be used during pregnancy or on children.

Essential oil of parsley is obtained from the leaves and roots of the herb, but mainly the fruits or seeds as they contain a higher percentage of essential oil. The oil is pale yellow/green in colour with an aroma similar to that of fresh parsley.

Parsley has been known about for centuries, both for its culinary use and its medicinal properties. The curly leaved parsley was popular in medieval England and connected with many superstitions and stories of black magic. It is meant to be bad luck to transplant a parsley plant, as old stories tell of its trip to see the devil and back, which is why it takes so long to germinate. It is also said only to grow where the woman of the house wears the trousers... The Romans made great use of parsley in their feasts and during merry making, to absorb fumes and avoid intoxication, the Greeks however, regarded parsley as a symbol of death and it was used in funeral rites.

Parsley is known to reduce fever, is a mild stimulant and a carminative. It has a tonic influence on smooth musculature, with particular influence on the pelvic organs and reproductive system. Its tonic effect has also been known to reduce broken veins. It has a reputation as a diuretic in the treatment of urinary tract conditions, rheumatism and arthritis. Spanish and French males say it increases their sexual prowess... they do eat a fair amount of garlic however, and parsley is also known as an effective breath freshener when fresh leaves are caten...

Patchouli - Pogostemon patchouli:
The patchouli plant is cultivated in India and first became known in Britain in the early 19th century, when it was used to scent imported Indian shawls and textiles. These were exported to many parts of the world.

The oil is a deep reddish brown, with the same thick consistency as benzoin and myrrh. It has a strong, musty, oriental odour - and has been likened to a stale, strongly perfumed flower. It was extremely popular in the 1960's and is well known as the "hippy" odour, reminiscent of Indian clothes, beads and shawls. The odour is very long lasting, improves with age and is an excellent fixative. Because of this, only a very small amount is needed in a blend and do make sure that the odour is appreciated before you use it, as Patchouli is usually loved - or not. It is commonly used in eastern perfumes, and with Camphor, Patchouli gives Indian ink its characteristic smell.

It is reputeded to be an aphrodisiac and can have a powerful influence on some (not necessarily just those around in the '60's!), however it is not to everybody's taste and sandlewood can be used as a good alternative.

Patchouli oil is good for apathy, anxiety or depression, is a good nerve stimulant and is warming and strengthening in small doses. Rather like ginseng, a lot depends upon the state of mind of the individual. It can cause loss of appetite and lack of sleep in some, and in larger doses can be sedative.

Robert Tisserand says, "Patchouli does not close up and obstruct where there is a natural flow, constricting only where there is abnormal looseness", and goes on to suggest its use for diarrhoea or constipation, oedema, obesity, water retention or loose skin.

Its antiseptic, anti-inflammatory and mild bacterial actions help in treating skin disorders from acne to athletes foot.

Peppermint - Mentha piperita:

Peppermint oil is extracted from the leaves of the plant and is pale yellow in colour. It is cultivated in Europe and USA. The odour is initially very strong, also with a strong middle odour. It is cool and fresh and very "pepperminty". It is a strong oil and should be used with caution. Although excellent against nausea, unfortunately peppermint oil has to be avoided during pregnancy.

Peppermint is known as the classic stomach remedy, is refreshing in small quantities and is a general stimulant. In too high doses it can prevent sleep, so care should be taken unless you specifically wish to stay awake. It is the best known remedy for colic, nausea, diarrhoea, sluggish digestion or indigestion, and other stomach disorders because it is a powerful antispasmodic and has a particular influence on the muscles. It can also have a numbing effect and can help with neuralgia. A cold compress with peppermint oil can effectively relieve headaches. Like rosemary and basil it is a "cephalic", clearing and refreshing the mind, and due to its instantly strong odour, peppermint oil can be used to relieve nausea or faintness by simple inhalation from the bottle or from a drop on a handkerchief. Because of its strong odour, it can offend, so care should be taken. Patricia Davis recommends its use against four and six legged vermin, placing a few drops on their runs to deter visits.

It also has a cooling effect in feverish conditions, and can cleanse and decongest the skin of impurities. For colds, influenza and the onset of feverishness, the warming properties of peppermint can stimulate and decongest. Dr Valnet recommends its use for impotence, although I have not heard of any case studies backing up this claim - yet!

Petitgrain - Citrus bigaradia and vulgaris/Citrus aurantum (amara):

Petitgrain or Pettigrain essential oil is extracted from the leaves and twigs of the bitter orange tree. As with the majority of citrus oils, the best is cultivated around the Mediterranean. Originally, it was extracted from the unripened, small fruits or "petit grains", before this became too costly.

The oil is similar to that of neroli, but is more refreshing and light. This gives benefit to a heavier blend where more pronounced lighter influence is required, as petitgrain is a very neutral oil. It is far less expensive than neroli and is also very popular due to its light, cleansing aroma. As with nearly all citrus oils, petitgrain is volatile and does not last long.

Rose/Rose otto - Rosa damascena:

Rose oil is the royal in aromatherapy and is quite simply adored by some. It is the queen of all essential oils as jasmine is the king. It is highly perfumed, highly prized and costly to produce. It was also probably the first essential oil ever to be distilled. Roses were used extensively by the Romans and historically, the oil was recorded in Persia in the 10th century. In Elizabethan times, scented food was very popular and rose petals were used for their beauty and odour, in the kitchens, in pot pourri and in scented washing water. Roses have been used for their scent, their beauty and their therapeutic benefits for centuries.

The oil is extracted from the petals of the flower, hand picked at dawn, as the oil content decreases throughout the day. It takes one thousand rose blossoms to make one gram of oil, hence the price. The finest rose oil comes from Bulgaria, from the damask rose, although there are other varieties used in aromatherapy. The otto oil comes from the damask rose, the absolute coming from the above or the cabbage (rosa centifoliar). The odour of rose oil is intensely floral, sweet and rich and is strong at all levels. If you can afford it, any blend will benefit by including rose.

Rose is an emotionally healing oil, with specific affect on those who feel ill at ease, who feel guilt, grief, resentment, jealousy, are unsettled or unsure or unhappy with themselves. It has a subtle yet powerful effect on the whole system, vascular, digestive and nervous, can regulate female functions, sexual difficulties and be a gentle tonic for liver and gall bladder conditions. It is the least toxic of all oils and is particularly beneficial for treating all skin conditions due to its subtle toning and soothing qualities. The planet of Venus governs the rose, its feminine quality having a definite affinity with the female reproductive system, in balancing, regulating and toning.

Marguerite Maury wrote: "As a well-known aphrodisiac, it is used in the Hindu pharmacopoeia reinforced with sandalwood. Our own experiences have taught us that the rose has a considerable influence on the female sexual organs. Not by stimulus, but on the contrary, by cleansing and regulating their functions. We have been able to test its influence on cardiac rhythm and blood circulation. The capillaries - those little hearts with independent beats - become active once more, and capillaropathy, with its sometimes tragic consequences, can be perfectly cured."

The profoundly positive effect of rose oil on the emotions, can be related to its influences on the female productive organs. So often irregular or scanty periods, infertility and associated menstrual conditions are related to a disturbed emotional level. There are many essential oils that have specific action and a therapeutic affinity with particular organs of the body, but none more so than rose in the realm of reproduction and sexuality. Rose is also particularly effective for skin care. Avoid using rose when pregnant unless under the supervision of a professional aromatherapist or if specifically directed in the A–Z.

Rosemary - Rosmarinus officinalis:
Rosemary is known as a symbol of remembrance, fidelity and friendship, is surrounded by tradition and legend and has many medicinal and cosmetic uses. The essential oil is extracted from the leaves of the herb, is cultivated in Spain and Tunisia and is clear in colour. The odour is fresh, cleansing and herbaceous, with a very strong top and middle note. Some aromatic constituents present in the plant do not exist

in the oil and the plant and the oil smell quite different. It blends well with tea tree and eucalyptus because of the high pineol and cineol content.

Rosemary is an effective general stimulant. It has a fortifying influence on the central nervous system, and is used in cases of loss or reduction in function or senses. It helps revive poor memory, the brain being the most vital part of the central nervous system. Greek students reportedly wore garlands of it in their hair whilst taking examinations (it certainly helped me during my exams, although I only used the oil - not the garland). It is good for mental fatigue and eases joint and muscle aches and pains. Rosemary is a fortifying and strengthening oil, and can help with circulation problems. It also has a therapeutic action on the liver and gall bladder.

Rosemary is an excellent tonic and is also good for any hair troubles, including hair lice, having a fortifying action when rubbed into the scalp. Rosemary oil is also good for general fatigue in children, or weakness during or after illness. Avoid the use of Rosemary during pregnancy.

Rosewood - Aniba rosaedora:
Rosewood oil comes from the wood chippings of the tall rosewood tree, grown in Brazil and South American rainforests. Rosewood takes decades to grow and mature and although it has long been harvested in the wild in Brazil, there has been no programme of replanting. This, along with other factors, is leading to concern over future supply. Rosewood is clear or pale yellow in colour and is refreshing, woody and floral. It is a gentle, neutral oil and although does not have a markedly therapeutic effect, it is a gentle tonic without being a stimulant and should not be underestimated. It is especially effective after "the night before", for clearing the head, and is particularly inobtrusive either on its own or in a blend with other, more specific oils. Rosewood can gently help relieve the effects of tiredness, nervousness and stress. Maggie Tisserand recommends rosewood for clearing the atmosphere, recharging your batteries and scenting rooms. Rosewood is not an overpowering oil, and a few drops on the carpet or in the hoover bag will scent a room without being too overpowering. It has a

gentle yet positive effect and is of particular benefit during pregnancy.

Sage - Salvia officinalis:
Although a favorite of Dr Valnet which can be a very useful oil for pregnancy and childbirth, this oil can be toxic in certain circumstances and should be strictly avoided unless under the treatment of a fully qualified aromatherapist. It is not for home use.

Sandalwood - Santalum album:
Oil of sandalwood comes from the wood of the sandalwood tree. It is cultivated in Mysore and India and is pale yellow in colour. The odour has a strong middle and base note and is woody, round and sweet. The oil is a good fixative in a blend as it is very long lasting and warm. It has over 150 chemical compounds and thus blends well with other oils.

Sandalwood was used for furniture and for decorating temples due to its scent and ability to deter insects. It is used in Ayurvedic medicine, in incense and as perfume, and is a reputed aphrodisiac. It gives strength and is a good "lift" for those feeling weak. Dr Valnet recommends it for impotence. It is a good physical tonic, especially for the reproductive organs. It is effective for back pain related to kidneys and adrenals, and helps with pulmonary conditions due to its soothing and sedative properties. It is an effective antiseptic, and good for all skin types. It is particularly useful for teenage skin conditions, especially as its odour is not too feminine and shouldn't put off the males. The therapeutic use of sandalwood has also been shown to help in white blood cell production by its stimulation on the spleen. Its widespread and popular use as a perfume upholds its reputation as an aphrodisiac. For those who find patchouli somewhat overpowering, sandalwood makes a good substitute.

Tea Tree/Ti-Tree - Melaleuca alternifolia:
Tea Tree is grown in Australia and the oil is extracted from the leaves of the tree. It has a strong aroma and is very spicy, warm and fresh.

Tea Tree is invaluable to the aromatherapist in that it is highly antiseptic and antifungal. Tea tree is excellent in treating infection, especially fungal infections such as thrush and athletes foot. Tea Tree has many highly beneficial uses and every medicine cabinet should contain this oil. It has a unique chemistry in that it contains trace constituents not found anywhere else in nature. French doctors use tea tree frequently, due to its high antiseptic value. Its many uses include:

Skin:

Boils   Cold Sores
Spots   Insect Bites and Stings
Burns   Lice
Sunburn   Ringworm
Acne   Inflammation
Corns   Athletes Foot

Throat & Lungs:

Bronchial Congestion
Sinus Congestion

Mouth Ulcers
Sore Throats
Toothache
Infected Gums

Aches & Pains:

Muscular   Aches
Arthritic   Pains

Female Problems:

Thrush (Candida)
Monilia
Cystitis
Vaginitis

Any fungal conditions, urinary or sinus infections:

Part of the BOC group of companies, now uses *Bactigas* - Tea Tree oil in a carbon dioxide spray, to disinfect, deodorise and "invigorate" the air and the buildings of their office blocks and hotels. This has been shown to reduce staff sickness and apathy and also cuts down mildew and mould in the buildings, thus reducing maintenance costs. The positive publicity of the varied and many beneficial properties of tea tree oil has led to a highly increased demand and during the last ten years, production has increased from 10 tonnes per year, to 100 tonnes* and still increasing.

The International Journal of Aromatherapy - Autumn 1991. Volume 3 number 3.

Even though Tea Tree is highly antiseptic, anti-bacterial and anti-fungal, it is still non-toxic and safe to use. A study by Penfold in 1925 showed Tea Tree to be 12 times stronger than carbolic acid, the then universal standard for antiseptic substances. This led to further research, still being developed today.

Tea Tree is one of the most remarkable of nature's gifts to us, as a natural, non-toxic and safe medicine, and even now we are only just beginning to comprehend its secrets. It is interesting to note that New South Wales is the only place (thankfully), where both the potentially lethal Funnel Web Spider and the effective antidote of Tea Tree oil is found... extraordinary?

Thyme - Thymus vulgaris:
Although this oil has many uses, it is toxic in certain circumstances and should not be considered for home use.

Ylang Ylang - Cananga odorata:
This essential oil is extracted from the beautiful flower blossom of the ylang-ylang tree (pronounced "eelang"), cultivated in the Comores and Madagascar. The oil is pale yellow in colour and is very sweet, exotic and particularly heady. It has a strong high and middle note. Because of its very "heady" aroma, the use of ylang-ylang is not recommended on those prone to headaches.

Ylang-ylang is a soothing, sensual and aphrodisiac oil. It has a positive influence on emotional levels and acts as a good anti-depressant. It is effective against introversion, emotional coldness, anger and frustration and is recommended for frigidity and impotence, or for those with sexual debility. It is known as poor man's jasmine. Ylang-ylang oil is recommended by Dr Valnet for lowering blood pressure and tachycardia (over rapid heart rate). It is widely used in the perfume and cosmetic industries.

PART THREE

VIII

·········· ✛ ··········

A–Z of
Symptoms

Abdomen:

Pain in the abdomen can be atributed to any number of conditions, from constipation to PMT. Much pain or discomfort in the abdomen is as a result of stress or tension, all of which can be greatly helped by aromatherapy and the use of essential oils. The most beneficial treatment is by gentle massage, baths or compresses. As with all pain, if prolonged and in the same area, seek professional advice.

For stress related abdominal pain, and for children, use:

Roman Chamomile	4 drops (2)
Geranium	4 drops (1)
Patchouli	2 drops (1)

When pregnant use:

Rosewood	4 drops (2)
Orange/Petitgrain	4 drops (2)
Patchouli	2 drops (1)

For both formulas, dilute in 30 mls of carrier oil and gently massage the abdominal area in a clockwise direction following the direction food takes through the digestive system. Never massage within one hour after a meal. If necessary, use a compress placed over the abdomen, using either formula above, with the amount of oil as given in brackets added to one litre of warm water or chamomile tea.

For infantile colic, see *Colic*.

Abortion:

For whatever reason or need, abortion can be a traumatic experience involving countless emotions, from relief and sadness, to great conflict and guilt. Apart from the physical trauma and the upset in hormonal balance, the emotional consequences can be profound. For many, there is an essential need to grieve. Counselling may also be necessary to advise about the possibility of future foetal abnormality (if this is the reason for abortion), contraception advice, or for associated depression.. It is recommended to wait at least three months after an abortion before becoming pregnant once more.

As with all degrees of grief, sometimes the only thing that helps is love and comfort and understanding and time to go through the process. For many, the loving care given in a massage can release much sadness or conflict.

For depression and quiet grief use:

Rose	10 drops
Petitgrain	8 drops
Clary Sage	7 drops

For despair and guilt use:

Sandalwood	10 drops
Neroli	10 drops
Geranium	5 drops

The above in a 2½% dilution in 50mls of carrier oil.

Abscess:

This condition can be very painful, especially if in the breast. If self treatment does not relieve the condition quickly, seek professional help immediately, as an abscess in the breast can quickly lead to a more serious condition.

To ease the pain and reduce the heat and hardness, use:

German Chamomile	7 drops	Tea Tree	5 drops
Lavender	5 drops	Lavender	5 drops
Eucalyptus	2 drops	Roman Chamomile	5 drops

Use either one of the above in a compress. Add the oils to one litre of previously boiled, cooled water or chamomile tea and soak clean gauze or a sterilised flannel in the mixture. Cover the whole breast with the soaked cloth, and leave for 10 minutes. Repeat every 15 minutes until the condition improves. If no improvement is noted within a few hours, seek professional help. If breast feeding, don't forget to wash off the mixture before a feed.

Accidents: (Also see First Aid)

All children have accidents, some appearing more accident prone than others. Your general approach to accidents is important, as there is a fine line between preventing serious damage or injury and helping a child learn by experience. It is hard not to feel over protective and wishing to prevent the normal bumps and mishaps that inevitably occur. This is especially so after the first serious bump occurs, generally around about the time when first toddling about, and a lump appears almost as quickly as it does on a cartoon character. It can be alarming and frightening, but stay calm and reasuring, so your child will not pick up any fear or upset from you, no matter how you are feeling!

Every year at least one in five children has an accident serious enough to need the doctor or hospital treatment, and clearly you don't wish to add to these statistics. There are many things you can do to help prevent accidents, and much equipment is available as an aid to supervision, but not as a substitute.

Sharp trees, wobbly stools, steps and stairs are all for climbing, giving challenge and excitement, any thoughts about care forgotten in the excitement of reaching new heights of understanding and achievement. Once the lesson is learnt that "hot" can be a nasty experience, falling can hurt and bangs and bumps are generally a pain, they are beginning to learn, but also gaining all this new knowledge can still be a challenge and fun. Try not to deny them the experience, but do prevent the risk of serious injury. Children are remarkably resilient don't forget, and life at this stage is becoming much more interesting and intriguing, if also much more tiring for you! Sometimes, a heavy fall, or a quite nasty bump will not even be noticed (except by you!) apart from their rubbing the knocked area and saying "No!" to the offending object.

However, as with all injuries, never underestimate the damage, especially to the head area. If quite severe, stay calm and be a comfort to your child, as any fear from you will create a vicious circle of pain and alarm in her. Be aware of any notable changes in character, as shock can often have serious consequences, and if in any doubt whatsoever, take her to be checked by a professional straight away. Don't ever feel that it might be unnecessary to "bother" the doctor if *you* aren't sure about the seriousness, let a professional be sure - they do understand your concern.

As with all scrapes and cuts, make sure that the area is clean and free from dirt. Bathe the area with warm, previously boiled water to which you should add Lavender, Tea Tree or Lemon. To a cup of water, add 10 drops of Lavender, and 10 drops of Tea Tree. Both are healing and antiseptic, Lavender more for the calming, soothing and healing effect, and Tea Tree due to its highly effective ability to fight any infection. Cover the area with a plaster during playtime to prevent any further infection, but let the air reach the area as much as possible. Once a scab begins to appear, use more Lavender oil to prevent scarring.

For accidents such as bruises, burns etc., check under the relevant entry.

Acne/Oily Skin:

Acne Vulgaris or *Common Acne*, is one of the commonest forms of skin disease and is due to overactivity of the sebaceous glands producing an excess of sebum, this often causing blockage and infection. (See sebum) Although acne can occur at other times, particularly times of stress, it generally begins in puberty and is associated with increased hormones, in either male or female. It occurs mainly on the face, chest and back. Use:

Cypress, Myrrh, Juniper, Lemon, or Tea Tree at first sign, with Lavender or Chamomile to aid healing, reduce inflammation and prevent scarring.

One drop neat on the "spot", or, for a cream/lotion, use unperfumed and lanolin free aqueous cream, or Witch Hazel gel, which is more drying, all available from the chemist. To 50 mls, add:

Lemon	12 drops	Tea Tree	10 drops
Lavender	10 drops	Chamomile	10 drops
Juniper/Myrrh	5 drops	Cypress/Myrrh	5 drops

Acupuncture/Acupressure:
The history of Chinese medicine is well documented and basically unchanged in its general principles, the basis of acupuncture now being known by many. According to traditional acupuncture theory, when the perfect balance of the complimentary forces of *Yin* and *Yang* is disturbed, disease appears. This inner harmony, and continuous flow within the body is regulated by the free flow of *chi* or *qi*, or "life force" (literally, "air" or "breath"). The chi flows along channels known as meridian lines within the body, and the needles used in acupuncture, as with the finger pressure applied in acupressure, stimulate the various points along these energy pathways, affecting the relevant organ or function connected to the corresponding energy flow. These energy pathways or meridians, are completely different to those of the lymphatic, circulatory and nervous systems. There are 14 major meridians, 12 paired, two unpaired, half yin and half yang. Any blockage or disorder along these pathways results in disharmony within the associated organs, causing a disorder somewhere in the system. Likewise, a disorder in an organ may cause a symptom somewhere along the meridian, either superficially or internally, causing an interruption in the various functions of nourishing and defending the body. There are some 360 pressure points along these meridians, all interconnected, all being equally important to the harmonious function of the whole.

Acupuncture, acupressure, holistic aromatherapy, meditation and yoga are all widely used to cultivate a balance of mind, body and spirit, often with effective relief of pain, addiction and disease. Massage along these energy pathways, especially with essential oils, can stimulate and decongest, thus help to strengthen systems and avoid common ailments by cultivating this inner and outer balance, and to maintain or achieve the harmony from whence all health comes.

In China, acupuncture is used as an alternative to anaesthesia for some major operations, and although we are not at that stage in this country yet, acupuncture, acupressure, reflexology, aromatherapy, along with the many other forms of "alternative" medicine is increasingly practised in the west, with countless surveys reporting cures and improvements, (*Which?* survey, 1985). 1955 saw worldwide interest in Chinese traditional medicine leading to the Chinese Academy of TCM being set up as a major research institute afiliated to the Ministry of Public Health, and as interest rapidly increases, countless other institutes are researching and evaluating the role of complementary medicine in diagnosis, treatment and understanding of disease processes, this to meet the increasing demand for treatment and information.

Acute:
An acute condition, refers to rapid onset, severe symptoms and short duration, such as any severe pain or intense symptoms.

Afterbirth: (See Placenta)

Age and Ageing:
Ageing happens to us all, from day one, and there is nothing anyone or anything can do about it. But, there is a way to age beautifully and look and feel younger than most people of your years (many or otherwise!)

The most natural and the most pleasant, is the most positive way of looking younger. Who wants to (really) go through pain and trauma of surgery, injections of hormones or the countless other "miracles" that make millions and make us look younger, either temporarily or suddenly? - especially when there is an effective, natural and thoroughly pleasing way of achieving youth and beauty, from inside and outside influence.

We all know someone who is healthy and happy, has "inner glow", and epitomizes youth, being full of vitality and spark. There are others who are perhaps riddled with toxins from an unhealthy diet or lifestyle, are full of stress and tension and thoroughly miserable, and look twice their true age. Health and vitality come from inner harmony and ease, this being precisely where aromatherapy and essential oils have the most influence.

The main benefit of aromatherapy is that it can be such a beautiful treatment. The aromas are wondrous, the treatment is therapeutic and restorative, and the benefits of the comfort and relaxation gained from a massage are without question. A relaxed and healthy body can efficiently rid itself of accumulated toxins, and restore a healthy bloom to a weary system and skin.

Cellular regeneration is the key to health and beauty and this comes mostly from within. Of course there are many external factors which contribute to ageing, such as exposure to extremes of temperature, excess sunshine and cold drying winds to name but a few, but the skin being the largest organ of the body, reflects the condition of the whole system. Good physical condition helps to keep us mentally fit and alert - and a fit and active mind affects us physically. Go for peak potential whatever age you are, (or feel!)

For a nourishing base oil, make up the following:

Almond/Peach/Apricot	70ml
Jojoba	10ml
Avocado	10ml
Wheatgerm	10ml (100mls)

For help with wrinkles, use a 5% dilution in 30mls of carrier oil, preferably Peach, Apricot Kernel, or Hazelnut or the above for extra nourishment:

Neroli/Rose	10 drops
Lavender/Chamomile	10 drops
Geranium	5 drops
Frankinsence	4 drops

For dry skin:

Sandalwood	12 drops
Geranium	8 drops
Rosewood	3 drops
Rose	2 drops

For normal skin:

Lavender	11 drops
Sandalwood	8 drops
Ylang Ylang	4 drops
Geranium	2 drops

For mature skin:

Lavender	14 drops
Frankincense	8 drops
Neroli	3 drops

For oily skin:

Lemon	10 drops
Tea Tree	6 drops
Cypress	9 drops

For Extra Sensitive Skin:

Rosewood	12 drops
Neroil	6 drops
Rose/Jasmine	6 drops

Alcohol:

Drinking alcohol, either before conception or during pregnancy may affect your baby. Although many women choose not to take any alcohol at all during pregnancy, either through preference or necessity, an occasional glass of wine, beer or champagne is not going to have too much of an affect on either you or your baby. The greatest risk is during the first three months of pregnancy, however if you do enjoy the occasional drink, make it an absolute maximum of 4 units each week and not all at once.

The higher the intake of alcohol, the greater the risk however, and babies of women who drink heavily during pregnancy may suffer from "foetal alcohol syndrome". This extreme condition is seen only in babies whose mother's drink in excess of 10 units per day. This can result in retarded growth and development, kidney, heart and limb defects, and characteristic facial distortion. For alcoholics, there are nutrititional deficiencies caused by excess alcohol in the blood stream, including zinc and other mineral deficiency, clearly shown to affect the baby.

The recommended weekly intake of alcohol for men is 21 units and women 14 units, in both cases with two or three days without taking any at all. During pregnancy maximum four units per week, with four or five days without. "1 unit" of alcohol applies to a standard measure of wine, sherry, spirits, or half a pint of beer or cider, although the wine and the cider contain slightly more than 1 unit of alcohol. If you need a "lift", try the following:

For confidence:

Jasmine, Frankincense or Sandalwood.

For depression or anxiety:

Bergamot, Neroli, Geranium or Lavender.

For emotional exhaustion:

Rose, Geranium, Neroli or Frankincense.

For anger or mood swings:
Rosewood, Chamomile, Rose or Geranium.

During Pregnancy:
Neroli, Bergamot, Frankincense, Rosewood.

Use a 2% blend of 25 drops in total, to 50mls of carrier oil, or sniff a handkerchief with a few drops of any of your favourites from above.

Allergies and Hypersensitivity:
During pregnancy, be careful not to make any major changes in your diet or lifestyle. Most women develop particular likes and dislikes once pregnant, however these are normally due to extra sensitivity, especially in taste and smell. If you do give up a food, ensure that you replace it with a near nutritional equivalent.

Some sensitivity may also occur to cosmetics and toiletries, even to some essential oils. There are many products on the market claiming to be "pure essential oils", some already blended, some not, however, do avoid cheaper, synthetic products as these are more likely to cause an allergic reaction and will never give the therapeutic benefits that a natural oil will.

An allergy is a reaction to particular substances which provoke certain symptoms whenever they are encountered. These can be inhaled, ingested, from contact or by injection. In normal circumstances, antibodies in the bloodstream and tissues react to these antigens with no further imbalance caused, but in someone who is allergic to a substance, this can result in specific reaction, varying from hay fever and asthma to severe dermatitis, migraine, feeding problems and poor growth in babies and children.

An experiment at Dukes University Medical School, showed a rise in the level of histamine, the natural biochemical secreted during allergic reaction, when a substance to which one is allergic is smelled. The imbalance in the system caused by an allergy, is often as a result of "over-doing" or an excess of a particular substance, be it anything from food to pollen. Babies can develop an allergy to cows milk, especially when newly weaned from breast - this can frequently be substituted with soya milk, often leading to a gradual tolerance of cow's milk protein.

Children frequently develop allergies to food, and if we are what we eat, then our children are certainly what we feed them. Allergic reactions to wheat or sugar are particularly common in children and an alternative to bread and especially sugary "fizzy drinks" having to be sought. Many children have allergies or sensitivity to additives and pre-servatives, with a noticeable improvement shown once certain food and drink has been eliminated from the diet. Never overcompensate with the substituted food, as this can cause further imbalance.

The first approach in treating an allergy is to isolate the substance or substances causing the reaction. This can be done by consulting a specialist in allergies, by Applied Kiniesiology, gradual desensitisation or an elimination diet. Attempts to identify, or avoid certain foods might cause more distress than the symptoms, so care and understanding plays a major part. The doctor may rely on anti-histamines and ointments to reduce reactions, although as with many aller-gies, such as infantile eczema in babies, asthma in children, and hay fever as adults, many are outgrown as hormonal lev-els change. There are now NHS clinics in the UK dealing specifically with allergies. In aromatherapy, the initial approach is to balance the over-reaction in the system, and to calm the tensions and stress associated with allergic reaction.

For inflammation and dermal discomfort, use:

German Chamomile	8 drops
Lavender	8 drops
Rose	5 drops
Melissa	5 drops

This in a $2\frac{1}{2}$% dilution applied to the area one day on, one day off for 10 days. Leave for four days and repeat. Also add to bath water as all are anti-stress in addition to being anti-inflammatory, healing and soothing.

For stress and anxiety use:

Rose	8 drops
Clary Sage	6 drops

| Neroli | 6 drops |
| Sandalwood | 6 drops* |

Use in a 2½% dilution, the above in 50mls of carrier oil, as a body massage, paying particular attention to the spine. Use the blend in the bath also.

*If pregnant, substitute Melissa for Rose and Frankincense for Clary Sage.

Amenorrhoea:

Amenorrhoea is the term used for the absence or stopping of menstruation. Apart from before puberty, during pregnancy and often whilst breast feeding, amenhoroea can be due to a hormone imbalance, disorders of the hypothalmus, ovarian deficiency, anorexia nervosa or emotional imbalance. See under menstruation for relevant formula.

Analgesic:

An analgesic is a pain reliever, usually applied locally. Analgesic oils include Peppermint, Rosemary, Lavender, Chamomile, Geranium and Eucalyptus, although aromatherapy stimulates the body's own natural painkillers - see under Pain and Endorphins.

Anaphrodisiac:

An anaphrodisiac diminishes sexual desire, Marjoram being the most effective, however, avoid the use of marjoram when depressed. Fortunately, high libido and depression rarely apply at the same time...

Anger:

When full of anger, there is usually an abundance of energy rushing madly about, or lurking powerfully inside, ready to burst out and flatten somebody, or reduce them to a "gibbering wreck". This is best avoided, for clear reasons, and if it is you feeling anger, demand a massage. If that doesn't work, gently request a massage, and if that doesn't work either, have a bath - on your own!

Use on yourself or another: Chamomile, Rose or Jasmine, or Ylang-Ylang. If the mood keeps swinging between murder and tears, use Rose and Geranium, with Rosewood or Bergamot. (If pregnant, use Geranium three drops, Rosewood four drops.)

Antibiotics:

Antibiotics are used to treat infections caused by organisms sensitive to them, usually bacteria or fungi. However, although antibiotics can be extremely efficient in killing these not so friendly bacteria, they may also destroy groups of harmless, friendly bacteria naturally found in the body, and result in side effects such as other infections developing. Antibiotics can also effect the absorption of oral contraceptive pills, so do check with your GP as to the effectiveness of your contraception, if taking the pill along with any antibiotics. In laboratory tests, essential oils have been shown to be as powerful and effective as common antibiotic drugs such as *penicilin, chloramphenicol* and *streptomycin* etc.* The selective action of essential oils does not kill off the friendly bacteria, but promotes immunity by stimulating the body's own natural defences. Antibiotics should not be used for minor infections. A common side effect as a result of taking antibiotics is Thrush, and if susceptible, you should advise your doctor. *Acidopholus tablets*, available from a good chemist or herbalist, encourage the health balance between friendly and non-friendly bacteria, also being an aid to eliminating waste products from the system. *R. Tisserand interview, 31.7.87.

Antibodies:

Antibodies are produced in lymphoid tissue in response to the presence of any foreign or potentially dangerous substance in the body. This production is the basis of immunity and "allergy", thus protecting us from harm. Essential oils to help with immune deficiency and white blood cell production, include Lavender, Neroli, Sandalwood and Bergamot. (See Immunity).

Anti-depressant: (See Depression)

Anxiety:

Most anxiety can be allayed and soothed away by loving care -

a cuddle works wonders and so does an aromatherapy massage:

Use Rose, Neroli or Jasmine, Bergamot, Geranium, Lavender, Marjoram, Rosewood.

Lavender	12 drops
Geranium	8 drops
Rose, Neroli or Jasmine	3 drops*

    *If pregnant, use:

Melissa	12 drops
Frankincense	5 drops
Neroli	3 drops

For a baby or toddler, a gentle and reasurring foot massage can work wonders, especially if they are too agitated to enjoy a massage. Hold her foot between thumb and fingers and gently but firmly work the soles of the feet. This method is commonly used in child care all over the world, and is calming and comforting, apart from working wonders.

Apathy:

As above, only with a compassionate yet firm and positive touch, using the choice from below:

Grapefruit, Orange, Jasmine or Neroli, Basil or Rosemary, Clary Sage, Frankincense, Sandalwood

Orange/Grapefruit	10 drops
Rosemary/Basil	6 drops
Clary Sage	6 drops*
Jasmine	3 drops – in 50 mls

    *If pregnant, use:

Orange/Petitgrain	10 drops
Frankincense	6 drops
Sandalwood	6 drops
Neroli	3 drops – in 50 mls

A drop of any or a mix on a handkerchief, or added to the bath (not too hot) will give a "lift".

Aphrodisiac:

Feeling good if not great, about yourself and your partner, is one of the best aphrodisiacs. The sensitive, intuitive, and loving touch involved in loving and love making can initiate

the deepest sensual response. A sensual massage with someone you love, who has also surrended themselves to touch
and experience, opens up a whole world of new aquaintance,
delight, joy and often suprise. The translation of touch into
feeling and responses can release a whole new experience of
delight and fulfilment. Try the following:

Rosewood	10 drops	Rosewood	13 drops
Clary Sage	6 drops	Ylang Ylang	8 drops
Jasmine or Ylang-Ylang	9 drops	Jasmine	4 drops

If pregnant:

Frankincense	10 drops
Neroli	5 drops
Patchouli	3 drops

To create a sensuous atmosphere, sprinkle a few drops of
one of the above, or alternativley, try Rose, Patchouli or
Sandalwood. Try it, there are countless combinations, no two
quite the same...!

Appendicitis:

Appendicitis is still the most common emergency operation
for young people. Inflammation of the appendix causes pain
in the lower right hand side of the abdomen, fever and vomiting. There is danger of the appendix bursting if the inflammation is allowed to continue, leading to peritonitis of the whole
abdomen. If in any doubt that pain or symptoms may be due
to appendicitis, seek professional medical advice immediately.

Applied or Systematic Kinesiology/Touch for Health/ Muscle Testing:

"Systematic kinesiology is the science of testing muscle
response to gentle pressure to find where imbalances in function or energy blocks are located in the body, and offers ways
to resolve them.

It enables investigation without intrusion, access to the
body's "computers", and gives insight to the underlying
causes of health problems. Imbalances are gently rectified by
touch and acupressure massage, which stimulate circulation
and lymph flow, and with nutritional support.

In this way, energy balance is restored to the whole person mentally, physically and chemically. It encourages natural healing to take place and enhances a sense of well being in healthy people." - Brian H. Butler B.A.

Muscle testing is often used by aromatherapists in assisting in the choice of beneficial oils specifically chosen to balance certain health problems. If a certain muscle is weak in isolation, relating to a corresponding organ or area, essential oils are tested to strenghthen and balance the weakness. Some oils may strengthen more than others, thus using *AK*, specifically effective oils may be used. Once chosen and mixed, the synergistic blend is then tested again against the weak muscles, and if strengthened, a massage will be given to strengthen and balance the whole system.

Asthma: (Also see Allergies)

Asthma attacks can be precipitated by exposure to a large range of stimuli, including allergies, emotions, exercise, drugs, and infections. Asthma is a variable condition, as attacks can occur at any age, for many reasons. Although normally ocurring in early life, asthma attacks are commonly associated with allergies such as *Hay Fever* and *Eczema*. Relaxation and avoiding stress can help to avoid the frequency of attacks.

Use Marjoram, Frankincense, Lavender, Chamomile and Melissa. The circumstances of the attack need to be taken into consideration when choosing the blend, it being a good idea to have an appropriate blend already made up if attacks are commonly caused by similar circumstances. These oils are most gentle, yet effective - to soothe both physically and emotionally. Most allergic reactions can be effectively treated with oils of Chamomile and Melissa.

If your child has an attack, whatever happens, stay calm and reassuring. She will pick up on your anxiety, so no matter how heartbreaking or frightening it is to see someone you love fighting for breath, panic will make it worse, so stay calm and have a sniff of the blend yourself. Don't forget the *Rescue Remedy* if necessary.

Massage can be highly beneficial, giving the patient the reassurance, comfort and calm needed.

Lavender	10 drops
Frankincense	8 drops
Chamomile/Melissa	4 drops
Marjoram/Melissa	3 drops

Massage the above in 50mls of oil, in long, even, reassuring strokes up along the spine, over the shoulders and on the chest. Alternatively place one drop of each on a handkerchief and inhale to release tension and spasm as heat from steam inhalation is contra indicated during an asthma attack. Pifco have produced a nasal inhaler, following the success of their facial steamer, which vaporises the essential oils with a minimum of heat, so virtually no steam is produced. The inhaler also has a spout to direct the vapour via the mouth for chest and throat treatments.

Astringent:
Astringent oils can help with fluid retention and to tighten lax tissues. See Ageing, Oedema and skin recipies. Astringent oils include Cedarwood, Cypress, Frankincense, Juniper, Rose and Sandalwood.

Athlete's Foot:
Athlete's Foot, or *tinea pedis*, is a fungal infection of the skin between the toes. The fungus thrives in this warm, moist area, and great care should be taken to keep the infected area clean and as dry as possible. Athlete's foot is highly infectious and children often pick it up at swimming pools or gymnasiums, as with verruca's. It can spread easily, so always use a clean towel, and don't share, preferably drying the affected area with disposable kitchen paper. Cotton or wool is preferable next to the skin as it can breathe more than nylon or other man-made fibres and change for clean as often as possible, (never swap feet).

Use Tea Tree, Lavender or Cypress. If quite severe, use two drops of Tea Tree and one of Cypress to a teaspoon of carrier oil and dab with cotton wool between the toes and nails of the affected foot. As the white, damp and spongy skin begins to dry and flake away, change the treatment to two drops of Tea Tree and one drop of Lavender, this helping to prevent the infernal itching as it heals.

Aura:

Most people know what is meant by an aura of well-being, yet an aura is often known as an energy field, seen by some in different colours signifying different moods and characters of people. The haloes depicted in religious art possibly signify the aura as seen by some. Kirlian photography shows this energy surrounding every living thing, be it human, animal or plant. From this special "energy" photography, it is possible to see just how much energy is increased after using essential oils and aromatherapy. (The difference between the spectacular aura surrounding an organic vegetable in comparison to an ordinary, is quite substantial.) Some aromatherapists work on the aura, not just the physical body, soothing a "spiky" or harsh aura into calm, smooth and balanced energy, or rejuvenating a tired, sad or hopeless aura with a positive and energetic "hum". Most of us feel it, some see it, but don't forget about it, as it can affect us in many ways.

Back Pain:

Back pain accounts for a staggeringly high amount of lost production world wide. It also accounts for a staggeringly high amount of distressed and frustrated people, often in a lot of pain. Back pain is the most frequent complaint, "alternative" therapists deal with. The majority is due to strain, spasm and tension and the associated types of back pain such as lumbago, sciatica and fibrositis, but many suffer from physical reasons such as a slipped disc or a trapped nerve. The spine is highly important as it contains and protects the spinal cord, damage of which can cause paralysis and severe injury.

Massage and essential oils can bring wonderful relief for back pain and the associated tense muscles, especially before, during or after pregnancy. It is particularly common during pregnancy due to the added weight and strain on the muscles, weak or otherwise, and the softening of the ligaments supporting the spine. As pregnancy advances, there is a quite natural tendency to over-compensate for the increasing weight of the womb by bending the body backwards. This c auses additional tensions, especially in the back and shoulders. If your shoulders are tense and tight, and you have backache, then you will not be breathing properly and will become more tense and tired and the vicious circle is created. No matter how impossible it may seem at times, if you *think* tall and light and relaxed, it *will* make a difference, and you will look and feel happier, lighter, more positive and on top of things instead of underneath the weight of everything. If you *think* heavy and tired and "elephant", your body will sag and will feel huge and heavy and more tired. If your posture is tense and heavy, and exhausted, then so are you.

Back pain, especially in the lower back, can be due to weak, under exercised muscles, especially of the abdomen, thus putting all the strain on the back muscles. Good posture and gentle stretching exercises can help. During pregnancy in particular, always bend yor knees when lifting or picking something up off the floor, and hold heavy things close to your body, (as close as possible!) Do not wear high heeled shoes, as this tips your pelvis further forward and puts even more pressure on your spine with the unevenly distributed weight. Try to do a few gentle stretching movements a couple of times each day, but avoid stretching upwards or bending forwards. Be aware of your posture as much as you can. Imagine a cord being pulled upwards from the top of your head, so avoid your head being compressed into your neck. Lengthen your spine. Relax your shoulders and drain the tension from them, including your neck and back, and prevent lower back strain by standing properly so that your pelvis is correctly placed and your buttocks and abdomen are supporting your lower back effectively.

If not pregnant, one of the best positions to ease backpain, is to lie on your back on the floor or a hard surface, out of draughts, with your knees bent enough to support the hollow of your back and your spine is fully supported - don't move for as long as possible! Whenever you get up, always roll on to your side and get up from all fours. This prevents any undue strain on your back again, and doesn't undo all the good work you have just done. If pregnant, lie on the bed, on your back if comfortable, with a pillow under your knees and feet, feet above your heart, and hips level (if you can remember where they once were!). If this position is uncomfortable, lie on your side, with your knees bent in the foetal position and a pillow under your top knee. Place a few drops of Neroli, Melissa or Rosewood on the pillow under your head, and relax with your unborn baby. Enjoy your time with each other and talk to her. You might even feel her stretching and relaxing and enjoying herself as well. Relax those muscles and breathe away any tension in your back or anywhere else. Close your eyes and enjoy the peace together!

Postnatal exercises can begin in the first days after birth, and are good for morale as well as your muscles. Often the pelvic muscles after birth are "out of shape", often resulting in difficulty in holding water, especially when laughing or moving suddenly. These exercises will all help. The idea of any exercise is not to make a pain or weakness worse, but to gradually increase the strength of the weak muscles and to increase strength and muscle tone in the area. If your back pain is frequent or incapacitating, check with your doctor or therapist first, to gain medical clearance, before embarking on any new form of exercise.

For general stimulation:

Rosemary/Lemongrass	10 drops
Lavender/Geranium	10 drops
Black Pepper/Peppermint	5 drops

For balance, harmony and bliss:

Geranium	10 drops
Frankincense	8 drops
Neroli/Orange	4 drops
Jasmine/Ylang Ylang	4 drops

For deep relaxation:

Lavender	10 drops
Benzoin	8 drops
Chamomile	4 drops
Melissa/Majoram	4 drops
(Neroli-optional	2 drops)

For a back massage during prenancy use:

Neroli   8 drops (or Petitgrain)
Frankincense   8 drops
Sandalwood   8 drops

The above in 50mls of carrier oil. Also add maximum 10 drops of a favourite blend to bath water for a soothing, pain relieving soak.

When manipulation to the spine is necessary, a massage both before and after treatment is often given. This relaxes the area before stretching and manipulation and soothes away any soreness afterwards.

Babymoon and Bonding: (Also see birth)

I include the "Babymoon" here, as like a Honeymoon, it is the one time perhaps more than any other, that you should make as much time as possible to be with each other, loving, learning and sharing, especially so if your partner can be with you too. Learn about and get to know each other by being close. Not everyone finds this easy, as a lot depends on how well and happy and relaxed you and the baby are, in addition to how your partner feels, but this is a very special and magical time for all of you, so if possible, make the very most of it, so that you, your baby and your new family get off to the best possible start.

The first encounter with your baby can often be as intense for the father as it is for the mother. From the very first miraculous moment of birth, you feel and experience the amazing warmth and energy of a newborn human being against your skin. Your daughter joins you both, she lies against you within your arms, and you finally meet this warm, crumpled, quietly alert little being, for the very first time. It is then that extraordinary things can begin to happen. After the separation of delivery, there are now two of you, and once she opens her eyes and you begin to take in that sweet, delicate warmth and weight of her, the communication between you, that began with the simplest of things, touch, a whole new world is opened up to you both.

She smells the scent of her mother and her milk, she feels your skin and the air, texture and temperature, she can hear the sound of your voice as she hears "hello you", for the very first time - and she looks into your eyes and face as if she already knows you.

As soon after the birth as possible, is the time for the family to be alone together. This first hour is all important, cleaning mother and baby, weighing, even champagne and cups of tea and toast can all wait. After the first hour or so, and mother and baby have relaxed after all their hard work (!) and father can relax at long last... baby will probably settle into a long sleep. This first time together is where bonding begins, and is the time for meeting each other and new beginnings.

The new born baby knows her mother by smell. Aidan Macfarlane tested breastfed babies of two and six days old, and found that they preferred the breast pad of their own mother to a strange mother's pad, and also in preference to clean ones. ("Olfaction in the development of social preferences in the human neonate", *Parent Infant Interaction*, Ciba Symposium 33 Amsterdam Elsevier 1975)

Thankfully, these days it is not the norm to separate mother and child after birth, unless there are difficulties of course, and mothers do not have to lie waiting longingly for their babies to be returned to them when it complies with hospital routine. There are many hospitals that provide a warm and loving environment, not only for delivering a baby, but for giving birth to a family. Create your own environment for birth by using essential oils in the birth room, not forgetting the oils for use before, during and afterwards.

Bach Flower Remedies:

Bach flower remedies have been effectively used by professionals and lay people throughout the world for more than 50 years. Dr Edward Bach, Physician, Homeopath, Consultant Bacteriologist and Harley Street specialist perfected his life's work of discovering and developing 38 non-poisonous wild flower remedies for countless ailments and conditions, both physical and psychological. Each remedy is correlated to individual temperament, personality or mood, to establish harmony of physical and mental equilibrium.

Dr Bach was an "orthodox professional" with great sensitivity of purpose and true concern for his patients, eventually giving up his lucrative practice to fulfil his quest for the natural healing qualities found in Nature. The flowers are steeped in spring water until the energies flow into the water. They are either used neat as in the classic Rescue Remedy, or diluted in water or liquid. They are mostly preserved in brandy and spring water. As in aromatherapy, an intimate knowledge of each remedy is required to match to each individual need, as no two conditions or individuals are the same.

Rescue Remedy is the classic flower remedy and is probably the most well known. It is a composite of five of the remedies - Star of Bethlehem for shock, Rock Rose for terror, Impatiens for tension, Cherry Plum for desperation and Clematis for bemusement. A must for every household, Rescue Remedy is invaluable in an emergency, for shock, angst or in any stressful condition, either as a preventative, during, or after. It is especially beneficial during labour and afterwards, when any dramatic shift in emotions or energy might affect baby's own natural equilibrium.

As with essential oils, Bach flower remedies can do much to help with the various degrees of emotions, from whichever end of the scale of feelings involved, for women in pregnancy, when giving birth and motherhood, for children and fathers alike.

Both essential oils and flower remedies are gifts from Nature and their effectiveness says it all.

Bathing:

Do not add essential oils to the bath for babies or children up to the age of 14 years old, unless under strict supervision and the oils are well diluted. The oil could irritate delicate mucous membranes, especially if splashed into their eyes.

There is no need to bath baby every day, especially in the first few weeks of life, as this can be drying to her skin. Her skin also needs to adjust to being out of fluid, and may react to being "outside" by being dry and flaky. (See skin care) On days when you don't give her a bath, top and tail her, by using cotton wool and warm water for her face, using a separate piece for each eye and cooled, previously boiled water.

Although there is conflict over the direction in which to wipe, the general consensus is away from the nose up until six months old, and towards the nose thereafter. When washing around the genitals, wipe front to back for girls. How often you bath usually depends on how often your baby likes it. Our daughter came in with us, "en famille", within the first week, and has loved it ever since, as have we. As long as she is warm, the water is not too hot or too cold, and she feels secure, she should love it, apart from the hair wash - which is normal! Most babies are happier in warmer water than often thought. Also, deep water helps to support them, as long as you ensure you are holding them securely – placing one hand on their tummy also has a calming influence (who likes a bath in 1" of tepid water?) If your baby does not like being washed in the bath, top and tail, and use bath time for enjoyment only, holding her close to you, until she gains more confidence and learns to like it. Once older, and toddling about, especially in the garden, a daily bath is much more necessary.

For you, a daily soak with essential oils is probably the most luxurious and delightful thing - and most necessary. Babies and children are in bed, and this time is just for you - enjoy.

For a relaxing, anti-stress soak, use:

Rose	3 drops
Frankincense	2 drops
Lavender	2 drops

For a reviving and re-energising bath, use:

Geranium	3 drops
Rosemary	3 drops
Rosewood	2 drops

For a sensual soak with or without partner, use:

Clary Sage	3 drops
Ylang-Ylang/Jasmine	2 drops
Geranium	2 drops

For a relaxing bath whilst pregnant, for both of you, use:

Rosewood	3 drops
Lavender /Frankincense	2 drops
Neroli	2 drops

Bed:

Bed should be a wonderful place, in which to relax, snuggle, enjoy, and have wonderful, healing dreams. A drop of your favourite oil or oils can enhance whatever mood you wish to create - see appopriate entry! In baby's room, for treatment of various common ailments or to ensure that the air is free from any airborne bacteria, place a bowl of steaming water on the floor and away from your baby, thus preventing her from concentrated inhalation, and add the appropriate oils.

Make her room a good place for her to be, with nice associations - she will then hopefully appreciate her bed, and "her time" (even sleep if you're lucky!).

Birth: (Also see Babymoon, Episiotomy and Perineal Massage)

During birth, all contact with the mother should be guided by her, and don't be suprised if instructions are short and not always sweet! Bear with her...!! The massage should be totally guided by her, what degree of pressure and where. Generally, a slow, rhythmic but firm action is the most helpful.

Massage around the lower back is of great benefit, especially with Jasmine, Neroli, Geranium, Clary Sage, Rose or Lavender, all of which have given wonderful results. For a back massage, lean or squat over a chair back, bean bag or the bed, well supported by cushions and pillows. Adopt a position of relaxation that gives you the control and choices that you need. You will probably wish to move around a lot during labour to find the right position at the right time. Use of the oils and massage, or of a flannel used as a compress, will also give your partner a much needed role. The sense of smell is particularly heightened during pregnancy and labour, (as are most senses!), so use your favourite oils to relax and soothe, which will also make the atmosphere more gentle and create a happy place in which to welcome your baby.

Aromatherapist Jane Atkinson has integrated her skills into the orthodox system at the James Paget Hospital in Great Yarmouth, by using aromatherapy to help women in labour – with great success (1). Women have avoided the need for pain killers – pethedine or epidurals, which is good news for both mother and baby, as although often highly effective, and they most definitely have their place, these can sometimes suppress function in baby and also "dope" the mother to the extent that she is not fully participating in the birth. No matter what pain you are going through, it *will* end, but whatever plans you may have had for your labour, be flexible for your baby and your own sake. Each pregnancy and labour is unique. Don't suffer unnecessarily – ask for help if you need it. Everyone is there to help you and help your baby into the world, and properly administered, pain relief can help "nip the top off" the peak of the pain, without your being totally cushioned against feeling. There are many midwives using essential oils with great success, and as more and more positive results are being recorded, more and more are attending courses to learn about aromatherapy, increase their knowledge or develop their skills further.

A stress free atmosphere and being able to relax as much as possible, is essential during labour, as high anxiety levels will block the release of endorphins, nature's own pain relief. Think "give" birth, and open up, not so much push and strain and remember that everything you are doing and going through is helping your son or daughter on his or her way into life, and into your arms. Ylang Ylang can also be of great help, although the headiness of the oil may be too strong for some, especially in the hot and usually stuffy atmosphere of a birthing room. (It has to be warm for baby, even though you may be dying in the heat – not everyone is working as hard as you are!). Jasmine or Rose, with Clary Sage and Geranium or Frankincense are usually more popular, added to their benefits of aiding the action of the uterine muscles, helping to expel the placenta efficiently, as an anti-depressant, for post natal depression and for helping to promote milk flow. Now is the time to use all the oils you had to avoid during pregnancy.

Warm, aromatic baths are extremely helpful and highly effective in relaxing muscles and easing stress both before and during labour, especially with the addition of suitable oils, preferably relaxing, fortifying and analgesic, to de-stress, give reassurance, strengthen contractions and so shorten labour. In addition to massage, essential oils added to a bowl of hot water, on the top of the radiator or sniffed from a hand-kerchief can also be of benefit in the labour room. The use of a burner is not recommended and will probably not be permitted, this due to inflammability of oxygen, cylinders of which are usually present.

Ethel Burns is a midwife at the John Radcliffe Maternity Hospital in Oxford. She is also a Clinical Specialist, Lecturer and Practicioner. With a group of interested midwives and the use of essential oils that would withstand scientific testing, along with "as rigorous a methodology as possible", they ran a pilot study for 6 months on the use of aromatheraphy and midwifery, the results of which are to be published in September '92. The project was funded by E.O.T.A. (see useful addresses)

Aromatherapy is well known in Germany, especially in midwifery, this as they were the first professionals to in-corporate aromatherapy in their state-run training courses. In Bavaria aromatherapy and homeopathy will be included in the examination for all trainee midwives from July 1993. (3)

(1) Nursing Times: February 27th 1991 – Theresa Swinnerton, Midwife.

(2 & 3) International Journal of Aromatheraphy: Spring 1992 Vol. 4 no. 1.

Blisters:
Benzoin essential oil helps to prevent blisters, also with Lavender to help heal them if they develop. If the blister is too full of fluid, prick it with a well sterilised needle first dipped into Tea Tree, then follow with Lavender to promote healing. A drop of Lavender on a plaster will help to heal and repair the damage, although as much air to the area as possible is by far the best.

Blues: (See Depression)

Bonding: (See Babymoon)

Braxton Hicks Contractions:

The uterus has practice contractions during pregnancy, in rehearsal for the real thing. These practice contractions are known as *Braxton Hicks* contractions and although often not noticed at all by some, they can often make you stop in your tracks and think "this is it!".

Breasts:

Once baby is born, sometimes even before, the pituitary gland secretes *prolactin* which stimulates the glands in the breasts to produce milk.

During the first few days after birth, a substance called *Colostrum* is produced, which contains all the antibodies and immunoglobulins which provide the extra immunity via you, until baby is capable of developing her own immunity. (See Immunity)

There is no doubt that breast is best for healthy immune functioning and new research published by the B.M.A. in June 1992 now confirms this. Babies fed on breast milk are more resilient and able to resist infection than those fed on formula. Many babies are also allergic to the protein in cow's milk, leading to diarrhoea, eczema and colic.

The sucking action of baby feeding from the breast also stimulates the release of oxytocin, which acts on the breast and uterine muscles, stimulating them to regain their former shape and position. If after-pains are quite severe, use Lavender and Marjoram as a compress.

Do please remember that if you are breast feeding, you must wash off all the essential oils to prevent baby ingesting any. Resume treatment immediately after a feed however, to gain maximum time and benefit - because initially you will be feeding very regularly and there won't be a lot of time betwen feeds...! "Kamillosan" ointment is highly effective, and safely avoids any further trauma of washing and drying to delicate and possibly sore nipples, as it does not need washing off before baby feeds. It is made from chamomile and babies seem to love it. A good friend who recommended it has always fancied it on toast, because she thinks it such a delicious smell, and no, she isn't pregnant again!

Feed baby on demand as much as is possible, then she will treat you more gently and not be angered or frustrated by the clash between your watch and her own body clock. Before a feed, empty your bladder and wash your hands, have a drink nearby as you can get quite thirsty and most of all, make sure you are going to be comfortable and warm, as if you are happy and relaxed, the milk will flow well. Baby should be warm too, although she will be warm snuggled up to you, and "fix" her to your breast making sure she is completely facing you, not just her head turned towards you, as the incorrect angle will not milk the breast and will pull the nipple and make you sore. Make sure most of the areola is in her mouth, not just the nipple. It will sound right when baby is swallowing, and feel right when it is comfortable. If you begin to feel sore, readjust baby, not your breast, gently releasing the suction with your little finger. Avoid clock watching and remember that the hind milk is richer than the milk that comes first, so let her feed until the first side seems empty - then swap sides. Try to start on the side you finished with last time. An easy way to remember, is to safety pin your strap to remind you, or when she is tiny and doesn't tend to wriggle about so much, lay her down on the appropriate side to start the next feed, but you should soon know which side you need to start on, by the feel of your breasts.

Relax and enjoy feeding your baby, you are both learning a new skill and a happy balance will soon come if you can persevere. Enjoy this precious time if you can, as it will soon pass.

To increase or balance milk production and flow, use:

Fennel	1 drop
Geranium	1 drop
Clary Sage	1 drop

(Equal amount of drops for a compress to cover the breasts.)

To tone, massage with exercise:

Lemongrass	10 drops
Geranium	5 drops
Clary Sage	5 drops (Massage in 30mls of oil)

For cracked nipples:

An effective and nourishing base oil to use for this condition is as follows:

Sweet Almond oil	90%
Wheatgerm/Jojoba	10%

Add to this base, Lavender and/or Melissa with Neroli, 2 - 3%, and roll the nipple gently between finger and thumb with the blend. Do this immediately after a feed to ensure as much benefit is gained from the blend as possible, and once feeding, "rotate" baby around the nipple, avoiding pressure on the same spot all the time. She won't mind as long as food is available!

For sore breasts:

Roman Chamomile	2
Geranium	2
Lavender	1 (Compress)

Let the air get to the skin as much as possible.

Also see Mastitis and Abscess.

Broken veins/capillaries: (See Thread Veins)

Bronchitis:

Essential oils and the use of aromatherapy is of particular use in bronchial conditions, as apart from the oils being absorbed into the system, they can be inhaled right to the centre of the trouble. The antiseptic properties of the oils, particularly Tea Tree, fight infection, the expectorant action of Eucalyptus for example, helps to expel mucus when the breathing becomes difficult, and the relaxant benefits of Lavender help with rapidness of breathing and shortness of breath.

At initial onset:

Tea Tree	2 drops
Eucalyptus	2 drops
Lavender	2 drops

Equal amounts in steam inhalation, or in room vaporisor (for children under five, only one drop of each). For over five's up to 14 year olds, chest and back massage also, as follows:

Tea Tree	5 drops
Sandalwood	5 drops
Eucalyptus	5 drops

In 50mls of oil. For over 14's and adults, double the above dosage and blend in 30mls of carrier oil - ie 5% dilution.

For associated coughs and chestiness:

Tea Tree	10 drops
Eucalyptus	10 drops
Lavender	10 drops

In 50mls of oil, massage chest and back.

Bruises:

Cold prevents any further damage to the living tissue beneath the skin, halting any further denaturation of the tissues. Immediately after a knock, the heat must be taken away from the area as soon as possible to prevent bruising. Avoid a hot bath after a knock, as even though a soothing bath may seem very appealing, it will make the bruising worse.

Use Lavender and Chamomile for their anti-inflammatory and healing effects. One drop of each on an ice cold flannel as a compress. In this case, homeopathic tincture of Arnica is invaluable.

Burns/Scalds:

As with all skin injuries, infection must be avoided at all costs. The severity of a burn depends on the area of tissue destroyed and the volume of plasma that leaks from the damaged capillaries. First degree burns involve damage to the outer or dead layer of skin, second degree affecting some living tissue and third degree burns destroy the whole skin thickness. Seek professional advice for all but the most trivial burns.

Immediately run the area under the cold tap or apply a cold compress to prevent the air from reaching the skin and to take the immediate pain away. Do not apply cream, oil or butter as this can lead to infection and keep the heat in. Apply neat Lavender to the area as soon as possible, avoiding as always the eye area. This will help prevent blistering or scarring and promote healing of damaged tissue. Lavender is also calmative and will help to soothe away the shock. Take a dose of *Rescue Remedy*.

If there is swelling, prepare a bowl of cold water to which you have added ice cubes, add three drops of Chamomile oil to a clean flannel or some gauze, rinse in the cold water and apply as a compress over the affected area. If infection does develop, use Tea Tree as above.

Candida Albicans: (See Thrush)

Cellulite:
Cellulite is the over accumulation of toxic waste, fat and fluids in tissue, commonly found in the thigh and buttocks and mostly in women. Skin in these areas becomes dull, with bulging and pitting resembling the surface of a mattress or orange peel and tissue examination would reveal the development of hard fibres in connective tissue. Deep massage of the area at this stage would produce a dull pain. Cellulite is common in those who under exercise, who are overweight or who do not eat a balanced diet, but whatever causes it, cellulite is an unsightly condition that can only be treated by a total programme of a de-toxifying diet, treatment and exercise, along with total commitment.

Lymphatic drainage using essential oils, (see *lymphatics*), combined with a suitable diet and exercise programme can help to improve the circulation necessary to rid cellulite. Rosemary and Basil are both cephalic, (clearing and stimulating), and Cypress and Juniper are both diuretic helping treat fluid retention and eliminate waste. Massage with these oils, along the affected areas, also take warm baths, (maximum 10 drops total in combination).

Chest: (See Decongestion)

Chickenpox:
Chickenpox is a highly infectious viral infection, the same virus being responsible for *Shingles*. The incubation period is usually two weeks, whereupon a rash appears, then develops to blisters and scabs. It can be distressing for a child as the spots are itchy and tempting to pick at. The patient should be isolated until the last scab goes.

As always, with any infection, sleep and rest is the best cure, helping the body to use all its reserves to fight the invasion.

For five to 14 year olds, use:

Tea Tree	5 drops
Chamomile	5 drops
Lavender	5 drops
Bergamot	5 drops

Add the above blend to 50mls rose water or chamomile tea and mix well before each application as essential oils do not blend well in water. Use a soft paint brush to coat the area and reduce itching.

For a bath, preferable for those under 5 years use:

Lavender	2 drops
Bergamot	2 drops
Roman Chamomile	2 drops

Be extra careful not to let the water get near eyes.

Chilblains:

Chilblains are caused by a lack of circulation, usually in the feet, whereby the blood vessels contract in the cold, resulting in a lack of oxygen to the area. Chilblains are sore, itchy and numb, all at the same time. To improve the circulation in the area, rubefacient oils such as Geranium, Black Pepper, Rosemary, Cypress and Juniper are all effective. Make a blend of eight drops in two tablespoons of oil and apply to the area with gentle massage, for a minimum of five minutes twice daily. This blend will be preventative in addition to a treatment.

Geranium	4 drops
Rosemary	2 drops
Chamomile	2 drops
Black Pepper/Peppermint	1 drop

Chiropractic:

The British Chiropractors' Association defines this therapy as a 'branch of medicine specializing in the diagnosis and treatment of mechanical disorders of the joints, particulaly those of the spine, and their effects on the nervous system'.*

*The Alterntaive Dictionary of Symptoms and Cures – Dr Caroline M. Shreeve.

There is similarity between osteopathic and chiropractic theory, both disciplines regarding the body as self healing, the osteopathic theory placing emphasis on blood vessels and circulation, the latter theory more on nerves and organs. Osteopaths are less likely to use X-Rays, and more likely to use soft tissue techniques and more joint leverage. A chiropractor is more likely to use rapid pushing movements to correct misalignment in the target joint, their task being to free trapped nervous tissue and the consequent malfunction of nerves and muscles.

Many disorders respond well to this therapy, and as with osteopathy, an aromatherapy massage works well with and is of particular benefit alongside treatment.

Circulation:

Essential Oils are absorbed through the skin into the blood stream and circulated around the body and organs thanks to our circulatory systems. They are carried to the various parts in the body along with oxygen, food and nutrients, where they are broken down, assimilated, used and excreted. An aromatherapy massage is one of the most effective ways of stimulating the circulation and carrying the essential oils around the system.

Colds:

With any type of chesty infection, especially a cold, avoid all dairy produce as much as possible as it is mucus forming.

For beginning stages of a cold use:

Tea Tree	4 drops
Eucalyptus	4 drops
Peppermint	2 drops

Use in a bath, keep as warm as possible unless there is a fever, and go to bed. Also use the following, especially during the "thick" of it:

Tea Tree	2 drops
Lavender	2 drops
Eucalyptus	2 drops

Use as inhalation and room vaporisor.

For the above use the recommended dosage for the age of

your child. These formulae are not a preventative, as the immunity to various infections has to be built up and established, however, the above can considerably ease the discomfort accompanying colds.

Colic:

When a child is suffering from colic, it could be due to any number of reasons, and as with any prolonged pain in the same or a similar area, seek further help if the condition does not ease within 24 hours maximum.

Bergamot	1 drop	Lemongrass	1 drop
Lavender	1 drop	Neroli	1 drop

Use either on a compress over stomach.

For massage gently over abdomen in a clockwise direction, also at base of back and buttocks if necessary, use:

Lavender	5 drops	Melissa	5 drops
Chamomile	5 drops	Geranium	5 drops

Both in 30mls of carrier oil. (Also see abdomen)

Cold Sores:

For Cold Sores or Herpes Simplex, use at first onset:
Tea Tree neat on spot, (not children under 14), or:

Tea Tree	17 drops, plus
Geranium or Lavender	8 drops - use in blend of 50mls.

Constipation:

For constipation, the condition can be eased by gentle massage around the stomach area, always in a clockwise direction, following the direction of the large intestine. Also massage at the base of the back and around buttocks if necessary.

It is very important to eat correctly to avoid constipation, especially during pregnancy when there is added pressure on the digestive system along with other internal changes, and it may be less possible than before to take exercise. Iron therapy is commonly the cause of constipation during pregnancy, although it can sometimes have the opposite effect of causing diarrhoea. Progesterone has the effect of relaxing smooth muscle in the body, and apart from sometimes causing constipation, the increased levels during pregnancy can often lead to haemorrhoids, heartburn, varicose veins, (including vulval veins), and also affect the urethrea – see *Cystitis*.

Because of all this, constipation is very common during pregnancy, which is the one time you want to ensure all toxins and waste is expelled as soon as possible. To help prevent the condition, along with associated problems such as haemorrhoids, drink plenty of water and fruit juices to reduce dehydration of stools, eat fruit and raw vegetables, not forgetting nature's own laxatives such as prunes and figs. If breastfeeding, do be aware of the possible effect on breastmilk and baby, so don't ever overdo it. Squatting on the floor or over the lavatory is a great help, along with deep breathing.

Avoiding constipation is particularly important if perineal sutures or a Caesarean section have been necessary, and any undue strain could cause distress. If you do have perineal sutures, hold the suture line with one or two fingers covered in clean tissue, to give support and "security" during defecation. It may feel as though all your insides are liable to fall out, but the chances are minimal... Don't worry if there is a small amount of fresh bleeding, as this is quite common, but do check with you GP or midwife if it persists. Chemical laxatives should also be avoided.

Marjoram	10 (2)	Rosemary	10 drops (2)
Rosemary	10 (2)	Patchouli	10 drops (2)
Patchouli	5 (1)	Fennel/Juniper	5 drops (1)

Massage in 50mls of carrier oil – drops in brackets refer to amounts recommended for use as a compress.

If pregnant, massage back and buttocks and outer thighs only and use:

Rosewood	10 drops
Melissa/Neroli	8 drops
Patchouli	8 drops

Contractions: (See Birth)

Convalescence: (See Babymoon)

Coughs:

Depending on whether they are dry and tickly or loose with *mucous*, very often a cough can affect the stomach, causing sickness, also the throat and lungs. (See *bronchitis and colds*). Massage the chest, throat and upper back with a blend of the following:

If very loose:

Eucalyptus	5 drops
Cypress	5 drops - use in 25 mls

If dry and spasmodic:

Lavender	5 drops
Sandalwood	2 drops
Eucalyptus	2 drops - use in 25 mls

Cracked Nipples: (See Breast Feeding)

Cradle Cap:

Cradle Cap is the term for the formation of crusty patches on the baby's scalp, due to an excess of sebum. It is very common in babies, although unsightly. Pimples form on the baby's face and scalp due to overproduction of sebum, which can sometimes form these crusts on the scalp. Never try to pick off the crusts, but soften them with the blends recommended below.

Blend one drop of Geranium and one drop of Eucalyptus with 3 tablespoons of sweet almond oil, massage well into the scalp. Rub gently with a flannel, or brush with a soft baby brush, in all cases avoiding pressure on the fontanelle. To remove, shampoo the head before adding water, massage in, and thoroughly rinse off in the normal way, taking care to avoid the eyes. Regular gentle brushing with a soft brush will help flake off crusts.

Cramp:

Cramp during pregnancy is often caused by the position of the baby, or by a vitamin or mineral deficiency, such as calcium or sodium. Circulation restrictions can cause cramp, which is often worse when in bed or towards the end of the pregnancy, when there is added pressure on circulation and just about everywhere else, as space becomes minimal. A foot bath and a leg and foot massage can often help considerably.

Use either:

Lavender	6 drops
Geranium	6 drops
Cypress	2 drops

or:

Chamomile	6 drops
Marjoram	6 drops
Cypress	2 drops

When pregnant use:

Chamomile	6 drops
Geranium	2 drops
Cypress	1 drop

Add half the above to a bowl of warm water and soak away, or to 25mls of carrier oil and massage the legs and feet using upward movements towards the heart.

Crying:

Crying is nature's way of letting others know something is wrong, and is also a release of emotion. A baby's cry will be tuned exactly to her mother's ear, and at full pitch can be the most excruciating sound, precisely to get her to act. It is an extremely efficient system!

For whatever reason, try not to let crying get out of hand, allowing it to build up into complete rage or frustration - in you or your baby.

It's difficult to spoil a baby with love and care, and although babies are suprisingly smart at getting what they want, when they want it, as long as she is secure in the knowledge that if something is wrong, and she calls for you in the only way she knows how - and you come, then the problem is solved. There is a world of difference in a cry for attention and a cry from distress or pain. A content and secure baby is less likely to cry anyway, unless something is wrong. There is no harm in saying "no" from the beginning, as when she gets older and learns that you and she are separate people, she will want to test you to the limit - then it's your turn to cry!

For adults' frustration and distress:

Bergamot   6 drops
Frankincense   6 drops
Neroli/Jasmine   3 drops - use in 30mls of carrier.

Alternatively, sniff a few drops of your favorite "lift" on a handkerchief and sniff, along with breathing deeply and thinking of happy things.

Cystitis:

Cystitis is inflammation inside the bladder and is most often caused by bacterial germs that normally live in and around the bowel opening, entering the water passage (urethra), and bladder, where they multiply. This causes irritation in the lining of the normally germ free bladder and results in inflammation. The symptoms are usually a burning pain in the urethra when you need to pass water, which tends to be more frequent than usual - then not being able to pass water. The patient may also suffer from aches in the lower back or abdomen, and cloudy urine sometimes containing blood. In women, the entrances to the urethra, vagina and anus are all close together, bacteria can travel very easily, thus cystitis affects mostly women. It is rare for men or children to suffer from cystitis and if suspected, the sufferer should be referred to a doctor.

Although the most common cause is from bacterial germs, other causes include allergies to toiletries, a particularly sensitive bladder, or friction of the urethra during intercourse. Always seek professional help if the attacks are frequent or if they continue for a few days, particularly if you are pregnant. The infection can spread to the kidneys if not checked, and during pregnancy women are particularly at risk from kidney infection.

The prime concern is to flush out the germs in your bladder. Water is the best to drink and the minimum of half a pint every twenty minutes should begin to take effect as the germs are slowly diluted and flushed away. Barley water or bicarbonate of soda in water, (if you can stand it!), are both good to drink, as they restore alkaline balance. The discomfort will get easier as you drink more liquid. The pain and anxiety of an attack can be most distressing, but try to relax with some essential oil compresses over your abdomen and back, with some hot water bottles on top for comfort.

For a fully body massage to relieve stress and discomfort, or for massage over abdomen, hips and lower back, use a $2\frac{1}{2}$% dilution of either of the following:

Chamomile	*or*	Chamomile
Lavender		Bergamot
Cedarwood or Sandalwood		Fennel/Eucalyptus
(both in equal amounts)		

For a compress over lower back and stomach, use:

Chamomile	2 drops	Chamomile	2 drops
Sandalwood	2 drops *or*	Eucalyptus	2 drops

For regular baths, use a combination of any of the above, to a maximum of 10 drops.

Live yoghurt is reputed to counteract cystitis also, by maintaining a healthy intestinal flora, as do *Acidopholus* tablets. Regular use of essential oils, especially in the bath, and following the guidelines below should help prevent recurrence.

Drink plenty of liquids, preferably water, and pass water as often as possible, as "hanging on" can encourage an attack.

Always wipe yourself from front to back to prevent germs spreading from the anus.

Wash morning and night and don't use perfumed toiletries in the genital area.

Avoid wearing tight trousers or man-made fibres next to your skin.

If you have any doubt at all about symptoms or infection, seek professional advice.

Cytophylactic:
A cytophylactic essential oil is one that stimulates cell renewal and cell regrowth, these include Lavender, Neroli and Tea Tree in particular.

Dandruff: (See Hair)

Deodorants

Effective deodorising essential oils include, Bergamot, Clary Sage, Cypress, Eucalyptus, Lavender, Petitgrain and Rosewood.

Depression: (Also see Tranquilisers and Grief)

In our modern society, "depression" is unfortunately well known. Depression can include feelings of anger, frustration and hopelessness in addition to sadness and despondency. Whether post natal, caused by trauma, a build up of stress or a lack of support and care, the depressed person generally cannot "snap out of it", and needs time, support and understanding. Use the following essential oils in the bath or as a room vaporiser, or self massage over the *Solar Plexus*, but best of all, a comforting compassionate massage using the following in 50mls of carrier oil:

Bergamot	10 drops
Grapefruit or Lemon	5 drops
Clary Sage or Geranium	5 drops
Ylang Ylang or Neroli	5 drops

For grief related depression, see Grief.

When pregnant use:

Bergamot	10 drops
Neroli	5 drops
Frankincense	5 drops
Rosewood	5 drops

Dermal inflammation: (See Oedema)

Dermatitis: (See Eczema)

Detoxifying;

The natural process of the body's way of eliminating toxins and waste is essential to maintain health and well being. Any debris left behind in this perpetual cleaning up process, both inside and out, from cell renewal to undigested and assimilated foods, can result in a build up of toxins if not eliminated efficiently. This can cause anything from fatigue to arthritis. To help rid the body of toxins and impurities, a balanced and healthy diet rich in natural foods is vital. Avoid anything with "additives", and ensure that adequate exercise accompanies plenty of liquids to help stimulate excretion and flush out toxins. Aromatherapy massage helps to stimulate this elimination process, in particular along the spinal area.

Use:

Fennel	6 drops
Juniper	4 drops
Rose	2 drops
Rosemary	6 drops
Eucalyptus	4 drops
Geranium	2 drops
Lemongrass	6 drops
Grapefruit	4 drops
Patchouli	2 drops*

All in 25mls of carrier at 2–3%   *Use this formula if pregnant.

Diarrhoea:

This can be from a physical cause, from bacteria or viral infection, as a result of tension or stress, because of anxiety or fears, from an allergy, or even from falling in love... The main thing is for it not to continue for more than 24 hours, as dehydration can result, especially quickly in children.

Try to avoid food, and drink as much as possible to help the body flush out the impurities and to replace the lost fluids. Use a compress over the abdomen, adding the oils to water, Chamomile or Peppermint tea:

Chamomile	2 drops	*or:*	Lavender	2 drops
Juniper	2 drops		Patchouli	2 drops
Neroli	1 drop		Rose	1 drop

If pregnant use:

Patchouli	2 drops
Neroli or Petigrain	2 drops
Rosewood	1 drop

Dilation and Curettage:

A "D and C", as it is commonly known, is performed under general anaesthetic, and involves the dilatation of the cervix (neck of the uterus), and the lining or *endometrium* of the uterus is lightly scraped off using a *curette*. It is performed for a variety of reasons, but commonly after miscarriage or abortion to ensure no material remains to cause possible infection. Conception is common after a D & C, so ensure adequate contraception is used.

Disinfectants:

To effectively disinfect a room, to inhibit or kill germs and airborne bacteria, use the following oils in either a spray, a burner, on light bulb rings or on the radiator:

Tea Tree, Bergamot, Eucalyptus, Juniper, Lavender, Grapefruit, Lemon, Lemongrass.

Diuretic:

A diuretic increases the flow and production of urine and helps to flush out any impurities in the system. Use Juniper, Sandalwood, Chamomile, Fennel, Rosemary, Benzoin, Frankincense and Geranium, either in the bath (maximum 10 drops in total), or massage maximum 25 drops in 50mls of carrier oil. Avoid regular use of diuretics, either natural or otherwise.

Doctors:

Whether or not you agree with "Alternative", "Complementary" or "Orthodox", anything that can help someone towards good health is a good thing, and no matter what camp you are in, treatment should be complementary. The vast majority of Doctors really are human beings who do actually care a great deal, neither are the majority of "alternative" professionals "cranks"! Talk to him or her, and you might be pleasantly surprised. See if you can help each other. Many doctors are interested in anything that can help their patients (and ease their work load!) but co-operation with him or her is essential.

Dreams:

There is conjecture that pregnant ladies communicate with their unborn babies through dreams, and vice versa. Be this so or not, there is no doubt that the majority of pregnant women have very vivid dreams. These dreams can be varied and so interesting and colourful that one looks forward to sleep and the next instalment! On the other hand, some dreams during pregnancy can be frightening, morbid and disturbing, but this is quite common and is a natural way of working out fears, desires and anxieties whilst we sleep. Write your dreams down, there are many fascinating books available on dream interpretation, and if distressed, discuss your dreams and feelings with your midwife, doctor or other pregnant women.

If your dream patterns are beginning to interupt your sleep and interfere with your rest and relaxation, have a relaxing bath before bed, to which you have added two drops Neroli, two drops Melissa and one drop of Frankincense. Use the same proportion of oils in a massage too, adding Lavender if it helps you to sleep, plus a few drops of your favourite oil on or around the bed..

Drugs:
During the first trimester in particular, when baby is at her most vulnerable, it is wise to avoid all drugs. During pregnancy and also whilst breast feeding any drugs taken by the mother will have an affect on her baby. Any medicines that have to be taken should be kept to an absolute minimum, and the mother be under supervision of her doctor or midwife.

Dry Skin:
The natural lubricant of the skin is sebum, produced by the sebacious glands. A correct level of sebum production, helps to maintain a healthy skin by conserving the natural moisture on the top layer of skin, too little results in a dry skin, an excess leads to oily skin, blocked pores and spots. A hormone imbalance can often be linked to an imbalance in the production of sebum.

In addition to a lack of sebum, smoking, alcohol, unhealthy diet and extremes of temperature can all be highly drying for the skin. Essential oils of Rose, Geranium, Neroli,

Chamomile, and Lavender are all effective in helping to restore balance. See Age for appropriate recipies.

Dysmenorrhoea: (See menstruation and painful periods)

Earache:
In addition to infection, anything from a cold to poking something in the ear can cause earache, however always check to see if there is any infection, as if not investigated, this could lead to serious complication. To ease pain and discomfort, massage around neck, outer ear and jawline with Lavender and Roman Chamomile. If the doctor has checked the ear and there is no damage to the drum, with his agreement, a cotton wool plug (not too small), soaked in a blend of warm oil with one drop of either of the above oils should bring relief.

Eclampsia: (See Pre-eclampsia)

Eczema:
For Eczema, Dermatitis and Psoriasis also see Allergies. The following oils are of particular benefit:

Lavender	15 drops	*or:*	Bergamot	10 drops
German Chamomile	5 drops		Lavender	10 drops
Melissa	5 drops		Geranium	5 drops

Use in 50 mls of carrier oil.

Always try a skin test 24 hours before use, to test for reaction.

Emmenagogue:
An emmenagogue encourages menstruation. These oils include Clary Sage, Peppermint, Rose, Fennel, Rosemary, Basil, Juniper, Myrrh and Marjoram. As stated, these are amongst those to be avoided during pregnancy. See Menstruation for further detail.

Endocrine glands:
Endocrine glands include the Pituitary (endorphins), Thyroid (governing metabolic rate), Adrenals and Thymus (governing the immune system), part of the Pancreas (regulating blood

sugar), the Ovaries, Testes and the Placenta, (hormones to regulate the maintenance of pregnancy). They are ductless glands, and secrete their hormones directly into the bloodstream.

Aromatherapy can work together with these chief balancers of the body, to influence and harmonise the complex functions of every system. Gattcfossé, the French chemist who first used the term *Aromatherapie*, classified the way the essences affect the endocrine glands and also how the nose and skin conducted the benefits of the oils to parts of the body.

Endometrium:

This is the mucous membrane lining of the uterus, which becomes thicker and richer in blood supply towards the end of the menstrual cycle, in preparation for implantation of the embryo. If this does not occur, much of the endometrium breaks down and is shed during menstruation.

Endometriosis:

This condition is when the presence of tissue similar to that of the lining of the uterus (see endometrium), travels to other parts of the pelvis and sometimes elsewhere in the body. The tissue undergoes similar periodic changes to the endometrium, causing severe pain and distress. These stray endometrial cells can attach themselves to any area, but more commonly around the ovaries, fallopian tubes and intestines. In many cases, endometriosis can cause infertility, the fallopian tubes and ovaries being surgically removed to prevent further pain and repeated surgery.

Recent research into the use of aromatherapy for endometriosis has shown that essential oils have a marked effect on the pain and stress caused by the condition. Endometriosis affects over two million women in Britain alone, and can cause immune deficiencies, hormonal, circulatory, lymphatic and cellular changes.

Aromatherapy can be of great help to sufferers, however always seek professional help from a fully qualified aromatherapist. Valerie Ann Worwood will soon have a book available for practical self help for endometriosis sufferers.

Endorphins:

Endorphins are nature's own pain killers, released in time of need. Don't forget that while you have this going for you during labour, your partner may be suffering in a different way, feeling helpless at "difficult times" for you, when someone he loves is in pain (and probably cutting off his blood supply by gripping him so tightly!). Have some oils ready for him too, for him to sniff from a handkerchief to give him strength and help. Essential oils are not strong analgesics as such, but they can effectively stimulate the production of the body's own natural pain killers. Use Sandalwood, Frankincense, Neroli or Bergamot - or for exhaustion, Rosemary, Bergamot, Lemongrass or Basil.

Episiotomy: (Also see Perineal Massage)

An episiotomy is a surgical incision into the tissues surrounding the vagina. It is most often necessary during delivery of a first baby and is carried out for one or more of the following reasons:

1. To prevent severe tearing or the mother has a fear of tearing.

2. Pelvic floor rigidity.

3. To hasten delivery. This may be due to fetal distress or complications.

4. Premature labour. If a baby is born prematurely, the bones in her skull will be softer and could be compressed by vaginal wall pressure.

Most tears that occur during birth, only affect the "superficial" layers of vagina and skin, they heal easily and are known as *first degree tears. Second degree tears* involve layers of skin and underlying muscle. A third degree tear is more serious in that not only are skin and perineal muscles involved, but also the anal sphincter muscle.

One of the most common reasons for an episiotomy is when forceps are needed to help baby into the world. This can often be an unnerving word to hear and they are certainly "off putting" to say the least, to look at, but try to think of forceps as protective, not destructive, to your baby, almost like a crash helmet if your imagination will stretch that far...!

Forceps prevent the delicate brain from pressure during delivery as they cradle the head. They may leave marks, but these will soon fade and disappear.

Perineal Massage has been used in many different cultures, in many different forms throughout history. This can help to avoid episiotomy and tearing. With more upright and active postures used during births today, a tear is much less likely, however it is a natural "hazard" of childbirth and is quite common with a first child. To avoid either a tear or an episiotomy, any relaxation exercise, in particular yogic exercise of the pelvic floor, can help to encourage the stretch of pelvic ligaments and relaxation of pelvic muscles. Warm baths and warm compresses also help to relax the perineal area, along with massage to stimulate circulation.

If stitches are necessary after the birth, use the following to heal and soothe:

In 1 litre of ice cold water, use:

Lavender	2 drops	*or*	Lavender	1 drop
Chamomile	1 drop		Neroli	1 drop
			Chamomile	1 drop

Mix the oils well, "swishing" the water just before you sit in it. Soak the area for a few minutes each day, or use as an ice cold compress as often as you feel necessary. Use of a bidet or the shower spray on cold, and on very gentle pressure can also bring relief, as can sitting on a rubber ring to ease pressure. Try to let the air get to the area as much as possible, using a hair dryer if necessary, as the dryer the area is, the quicker it will heal. A pillow between your knees when lying down will also help the air to circulate. Change pads as often as possible.

Exercise:

The somewhat self indulgence of the 1960's and '70's, led to the fitness revolution of the '80's, and a huge surge of interest and enthusiasm for physical fitness. There is no doubt that health and well-being can be improved by a balanced diet, exercise and a healthy lifestyle. Exercise is certainly not a universal panacea for all unhealthiness however, neither is it dangerous as long as it is performed correctly, especially if going all out to regain your shape after giving birth. Before embarking on any fitness program, especially if new to you and soon after birth, check with your GP to ensure it will be right for you.

Warm up is essential to loosen and stretch muscles and prevent injury in any exercise. Equally important is the "warm down", to prevent build up of lactic acid in the muscles and reduce stiffness. (A little stiffness shows you have worked the muscles and could certainly be fitter, but being unable to walk afterwards is completely over doing it.) Exercise can undoubtedly relieve stress, anxiety, depression, improve work and sexual performance, make you glow with health and beauty and make you live longer - however, there are pitfalls. Some quite serious injuries have been caused by over enthusiatic exercising, including damaged and torn muscles and tendons, impaired libido and fertility and even heart attacks.

Providing the exercise you take is performed in the right setting, with the right equipment, and you don't suddenly go at it like a maniac for instant results, you can avoid the risk of muscular injuries or potentially serious injury. Listen to your body, and if bits begin to creak or groan, ease off. "Going for the Burn", has now been established as the wrong way to do things. To become fit and fitter, you train your body and muscles to do more work with less effort - gradually. Sustained, regular exercise of a minimum of three, 30 - 40 minute exercise sessions, spaced through the week, will force the heart and lungs to work harder to supply muscles with oxygen, thus using energy and reducing excess weight. As your fitness level improves, you have to work harder for the same benefit, muscles become stronger and you gradually look and feel fitter and healthier. Never embark on a new form of exercise whilst pregnant without the full agreement of your doctor or midwife, and only if gentle. For before exercise, to stimulate circulation and to warm up those muscles, use:

Rosemary	10 drops
Lavender	8 drops
Grapefruit	5 drops
Black Pepper	2 drops - in 50mls.

For after exercise and to help eliminate any toxins, lactic acid build up and so help prevent stiff muscles, use:

Lavender	10 drops (5)
Petitgrain	6 drops (2)
Lemongrass	5 drops (2)
Juniper	4 drops (1) in 50mls, (also in the bath)

Exhaustion:

For exhaustion, either before, during or after... massage with either formula below; in 50mls (and in the bath), use:

Rosewood	10 drops (4)	Rosemary	8 drops (3)
Pettigrain	10 drops (4)	Geranium	8 drops (3)
Jasmine	5 drops (2)	Lavender	8 drops (2)

Expectorant:

An expectorant should aid the expulsion of phlegm/mucous. Expectorant essential oils include Bergamot, Eucalyptus, Benzoin, Marjoram, Sandalwood and Myrrh. (Also see under Bronchitis, colds etc.)

Experts:

There are those who claim to be, those who are, and those who should be. Never be put off or confused by The Experts, always ask if you aren't sure of anything, but whatever your opinion, always listen, because there is always something to learn and something which might help either you or your family.

Eyes:

Never use essential oils in or near the eyes as they can irritate delicate membranes. Newborn babies often have a "sticky" eye when born and the most effective and the most natural antidote, is *Colostrum*. Colostrum is the first "milk" produced, and is packed with all the antibodies she will need. A small "squirt" in the eye will work wonders for any eye problems baby may have. (Just as well they can't focus too well!)

Feet:

Our feet are not on view that often and if most of us were honest, our feet only get real attention if there is a problem - other

than that, it's usually a daily wash and an occasional pedi-
cure. During pregnancy, swollen ankles and feet are a very
common problem, especially during the afternoon or in
warmer weather. Avoid wearing high heels during pregnancy,
as apart from tipping your pelvis further forward, your
increasing weight is not evenly distributed. Try to wear "flat-
ties" throughout your pregnancy, to help maintain your posture and prevent aches and pains later on.

Love them or not, our feet are very important to us and
apart from having 72,000 nerve endings dotted about them,
they take a heck of a bashing one way or another! From birth
until maturity at about 17 years old, our feet are very supple
and can easily be distorted without any pain being caused.
The bones in a child's feet are particularly pliable and she will
not necessarily let you know if her shoes are too small or ill fitting, because it might not hurt her. The correct footwear is
essential and then only when feet and legs are strong enough
for walking. Don't encourage your child to walk before she is
ready and has sufficient balance and co-ordination. A newborn baby's stepping movements are due to one of the several
primitive reflexes we are born with, such as sucking, grasping
and so on. She has no real control over this 'stepping reflex'
and without your firm support would certainly collapse if you
let go. She needs time to build up strength and confidence at
each stage of development, to go happily and naturally on to
the next. All babies are different and as long as you and she
enjoy each stage of development, you can both happily go on
to learn about the next - and they keep coming, voluntarily or
otherwise!

Encourage your child to go barefoot as often as possible
(you too), without the restriction of shoes or socks - too tight
all-in-one suits or socks can be just as damaging as ill fitting
shoes. Baby's toes grip the floor naturally and help in balance
and at this stage she only really needs shoes for walking outside or for protection.

Keep feet clean and dry them thoroughly, especially
between the toes, as any area of warmth and moisture is an
ideal breeding ground for bacteria and infection. Toenails
should be cut across and never down at the corners. Careful

use of sharp nail clippers give a quick and clean cut. Some mothers bite their baby's nails, but I found this tended to leave an uneven edge, especially if your child has strong nails.

Children's shoes are expensive, especially for something so very small, but proper fitting facilities are usually only available at the more expensive shoe shops and the investment in your child's shoes, although they can only last for several weeks, is an investment to prevent damaged and distorted feet that could plague your child in later years. The shoes should be of adequate length, width, depth and ankle support. An ankle fastening is preferable to a slip-on, as this holds the shoe firmly on the foot, allowing it to work normally and not have to work to keep the shoe on.

If you do need to see a chiropodist or a reflexologist, do make sure they are properly registered. When pregnant, or you have a child under one, treatment and advice is available under the NHS for chiropody and the Chiropodist should be qualified with the letters "SRCh" or "MChs". Many chiropodists and reflexologists now use essential oils as part of their treatment.

A soothing foot massage with essential oils, is sheer delight after a long day, especially when pregnant and the poor old feet are carrying even more weight about. Again, try to avoid shoes as much as possible and if it isn't too cold, let them breathe as much as possible. Rest as much as you can, with your feet above your heart, you will be running about enough after baby is born, so make the most of it

For a Foot Massage and Footbath:

Refreshing:

Peppermint
Lemon/Grapefruit

For tired and swollen feet:

Chamomile
Bergamot

For improved circulation and to ease weariness:

Geranium
Fennel
Orange/Petitgrain

For specific foot problems such as verrucas, athletes foot etc., see relevant alphabetical entry.

Femininity:
When you feel like a great lump, it's hard to feel feminine, even though being pregnant is the most obvious sign of being a female! When baby is born, there is little time for you and even less to pamper yourself, but try to make time for you and yours. No matter how much you love your baby, and probably want to be with her and your partner for most of the time (often by necessity), try to give yourself a little space alone each day, at least your very own time in the bath. Bathe in the beauty and benefits of a luxurious aromatic bath with the more exotic essential oils, in particular those you had to avoid during pregnancy. Use Jasmine, Rose and Neroli for sheer luxury. Get to know yourself again, and the new you now you are a mother, and nourish and pamper yourself at least during bath time. If you feel good inside, and happy with yourself, that inside smile will shine outwads and even that once "svelt" (ish!) figure will soon return. You are how you feel, so do everything you can to feel good.

Fevers:
A febrifuge essential oil is one that helps to reduce or prevent fever, by lowering the body temperature. Febrifuge drugs include paracetamol and aspirin. Febrifuge essential oils include Bergamot, Chamomile, Melissa, Eucalyptus and Lavender.

When the body shivers, it is not necessarily due to coldness, but using natural resources to shake off the fever and reduce body temperature. To reduce temperature, sponge with lukewarm water to which essential oils have been added, especially on the back, this being the greatest overall expanse of skin area, also under the armpits, temples and wrists. A compress on the forehead or lower back can also help. Cold water is not recommended, as this makes the blood vessels contract in normal reaction to cold, thus keeping the heat in. Add two drops of essential oil to one litre of water. Peppermint may also be used in a room vaporiser. (See temperature.)

Flatulence:

Flatulence can be caused by overeating, or eating particularly gas-inducing foods. Unless it is a temporary problem a visit to a qualified nutritional adviser is recommended for possible change of diet. Essential oils to help, include Fennel and Peppermint, but not whilst pregnant. Added pressure on the internal organs during pregnancy can cause considerable discomfort, including palpitations, heartburn and flatulence. Either "upper" or "lower" wind can be exacerbated especially if not "released", so, not to put too finer point on it - let it go whenever you can. Always try to evacuate the bowels regularly to prevent a build up of gasses. When pregnant, use oils of Lemon and Bergamot as inhalants or in room difusers. Post natal "windiness" can be due to weakness of pelvic floor muscles so make sure you do your exercises!! (Also see constipation.)

Fluid Retention: (See Oedema)

Forceps: (See Episiotomy)

Frigidity:

Unlike impotence, frigidity in a female does not impair function, but pleasure - the woman often being unable to reach a peak of sexual fulfilment. She might have a lack of sexual desire, or even complete dislike of any sexual activity. Oils to use in cases of frigidity include the particularly feminine oils, such as Rose, to give confidence in womanhood and overcome anxiety; Ylang Ylang, to soothe and increase libido; Neroli to give a lift and release stress, and Jasmine to boost sensuality and heighten desire. These particular oils are elegant, sensual and exotic and a little more fortifying than Clary Sage or Sandalwood, but you will find your own preferences. Use in a massage with your partner, to soothe and calm the central nervous system, thus relaxing and soothing emotions and anxieties. Enjoy the massage and the benefits of the oils, and avoid thinking of any pressures of lovemaking, you are loving right now if relaxed and calm. The most beautiful love to be made is in the depth of caring and the warmth of true emotion, which can be shown in massage, a simple caress or even simply in the warmth of holding each other.

Fungi:
The most effective anti-fungal essential oil is Tea Tree oil. Other oils to inhibit the growth of moulds, fungi, yeasts etc., include Eucalyptus, Lavender and Myrrh. For specific remedies such as Athlete's foot etc., see relevant entry.

German Measles: (See Rubella)

Gingivitis:
More teeth are lost through gum disease than through tooth decay, gingivitis often leading to infection if not checked. Gingivitis is inflammation of the gums and is very common during pregnancy. Mouth hygiene is vital to prevent infection, although avoid unecessary and overuse of antiseptic mouth washes, many of which kill off friendly bacteria in addition to unfriendly. Whilst pregnant, keep teeth and gums clean by regular and correct brushing, and finger massage gums to encourage and stimulate circulation and health. Have dental checks regularly of course and don't forget that the service is (currently) free during pregnancy and for 12 months after the birth. If outside pregnancy, mouthwash with Fennel or Myrrh to strengthen, heal and give tone. If pregnant, use Tea Tree.

Grief:
Love and understanding can often be the simplest and most effective comfort for grief. Emotional consequences of grief can be profound, and depending on the degree, a time of grieving and consequent healing cannot and should not be avoided or hurried. Understanding and love can only help with this most natural of processes, helped by essential oils of Neroli, Rose (for past or recent grief), Benzoin and Jasmine.

Gums: (See Gingivitis)

Haemorrhoids:

Haemorrhoids, or piles as they are more frequently known, are common during pregnancy, this due to the added pressure on internal organs from the expanding uterus, constipation and the strain often involved in evacuating the bowels. (Also see Constipation, and the effect of progestegen on smooth muscle). Use two drops of Geranium and one drop of Cypress in a bowl of water and sit for as long as comfortable. Alternatively, add one drop of Geranium and one drop of Cypress to approximately one inch of KY Jelly or the equivalent amount of Vaseline or Aqueous cream and apply twice each day, particularly after a bowel movement. Ensure the area is clean and dry before application.

Hair:

For all the recipies below, the blend is based on 50mls of carrier oil. Massage the blend into the scalp and hair and leave for at least one hour, 2 to 3 times each week, depending on the degree of treatment required. To remove the blend, ensure that you work shampoo well into the scalp and hair *before* you add any water, as this helps to break down the oil before you are able to wash it out.

For dry hair:

| Rosewood | 15 drops |
| Sandalwood | 10 drops |

For oily hair:

| Bergamot | 12 drops |
| Lavender | 13 drops |

For dandruff:

| Eucalyptus | 10 drops |
| Rosemary | 15 drops |

To strengthen hair:

Rosemary	9 drops
Lavender	9 drops
Bergamot	7 drops

*For head lice/ticks

Tea Tree	25 drops
Geranium	15 drops
Eucalyptus	15 drops
Lavender	20 drops

* Use the above formula in 100 mls of carrier oil and massage well into scalp, hair and roots. Wrap the head in cling film to keep warm and leave on for at least one hour. Repeat every two days for a week to a maximum of 10 days. Repeat if necessary after two weeks.

Hands:

Hands are often neglected, even though they work so very hard for us in virtually everything we do. Much tension can accumulate in the hands, anxiousness and stress showing in clenched fists, bitten nails, finger drumming and hand wringing to name but few signs. They are very rarely still and relaxed, so a massage to stretch and release stress can ease much accumulated tension.

Hands can also become very dry, especially if neglected once baby comes along and they are immersed in water far more often than they were before. Add the following oils to cream to make a nourishing and rich hand cream for family use:

Benzoin, Lavender, Lemon, Chamomile in equal amounts, plus Rose or Orange Flower water if required. Bear in mind that if your hands are particularly sensitive, the classic anti-allergy oils are Chamomile and Melissa.

Hangover:

Of course this formula probably only applies to the family members who have celebrated your giving birth and the baby, but should it apply at any other time.... the same will apply:

Place one drop each, or separately, (depending how you feel!), of Rosewood or Rosemary on a handkerchief and inhale deeply, or add 3 drops of each to the bath. An alternative bath soak is:

Fennel   2 drops
Juniper   2 drops
Rosemary   1 drop

Eat something, drink lots of water and take the or any dog for a walk. If it's a real "humdinger", place a cold flannel soaked in Peppermint/Rosewood/Lavender over the temples, and go to bed before you talk to anyone!

Hayfever: (Also see Allergies)

In addition to the recommendations given under the "Allergy" entry, with particular reference to hayfever, there are some excellent Homeopathic remedies available as well as the aromatherapy below. The most common symptoms of hayfever are inflammation of the membrane lining of the nose and sometimes conjunctiva, leading to sneezing, running nose and watering eyes.

Approximately 10 million people suffer from hayfever in this country, a pollen count of only 50 grains per cubic metre of air being enough to provoke a sneeze. A human sneeze travels at over a hundred miles per hour, which is faster than the speed of a bullet, and if persistant, can be exhausting, so try Melissa, Chamomile, Lavender or Eucalyptus on a handkerchief to sniff.

Headaches:

Most headaches are stress related, some can be due to physical illness, others as a reaction to the environment and some precipitated by food allergy. In children too, the most common causes are due to lack of sleep, eye strain, (due to too much television or homework if you are lucky), or as a result of allergic reaction. Oral contraception can also cause headaches, this is due to the change in hormonal balance. You may need to change the strength or even the brand, so check with your GP.

Use essential oils of Grapefruit, Rosemary, Peppermint, Roman Chamomile or Neroli. Lavender essential oil is sometimes effective in easing headaches, but after initial relief, has been known to be associated with nausea*. Inhale one or two drops of oil from a handkerchief, or use a cool flannel as a compress over the forehead and temples, using four drops to one litre of water or chamomile/peppermint tea.*

Nursing Times, August 7th 1991: Marjorie Smith - Midwife and nurse in the children's wing at Leeds General Infirmary.

Healing/Health:

During labour and birth the immune system has taken quite a bashing one way or another. To stimulate the healing processes and boost the weakened system, massage the spinal area in particular, as the oils will be absorbed more rapidly via the central nervous system and promote healing and recovery. See relevant entry under Immunity etc..

Heat: (Bumps/Rash/Prickly - See Rashes)

Herbs: (Teas)

Coffee and tea should be avoided during pregnancy, as both contain varying amounts of caffeine, an addictive stimulant drug that can cause over activity of the nervous system. It can increase blood pressure and heart rate, and if drunk at meal times, can reduce the absorption of iron. De-caffinated tea or coffee is not a good substitute, this due to the chemicals used to extract the caffeine, all of which can cross the placenta to your baby.

There is now such a wide range of herbal teas available, there is certainly one that will compensate. Peppermint is an excellent drink to combat nausea, Chamomile is calming and soothing and Raspberry Leaf (taken in the last 2–4 weeks of pregnancy) is famous for helping to ease difficulties in labour.

Herpes:

The virus *Herpes Simplex* is often carried without any of the customary accompanying cold sores. They usually appear when the immune system is weak, or when the carrier is run-down, tired or stressed and resistance is low. A dab of neat Bergamot, Tea Tree or Lavender should be applied at the very first sign and continued in a teaspoonful of an alcohol base, (this is more drying than oil as a carrier). Buy alcohol from the chemist if possible, however if not available, the purest and most suitable alcohol to use which is readily available, is vodka.

Herpes Zoster occurs as Shingles in adults and can cause Chickenpox in children (see relevant entries). *Genital Herpes* is an extremely contagious sexually transmitted disease.

Hiccoughs:

The characteristic sound of a *"hiccup"* is caused by the involuntary and abrupt lowering of the diaphragm and the consequent closing of the upper end of the trachea as the breath is drawn in. They usually occur repeatedly for a minute or longer, but prolonged hiccoughs can be distressing, exhausting and often a sign of other disorders. If they persist for longer than 24 hours or are particularly distressing, seek medical advice. Sometimes pressure or finger massage behind the apesternal notch (the "dip" below the adam's apple), can relieve hiccoughs.

High Blood Pressure (Hypertension):
Aromatherapy massage can most certainly help with high blood pressure, even more so when in conjunction with changes and improvements to diet and lifestyle.

Hypertension or high blood pressure, should reduce naturally under normal conditions, however if continued, could lead to more serious conditions affecting the arteries, such as arteriosclerosis and atheroma, limiting blood circulation and possibly leading to thrombosis and thus increasing the likelyhood of a stroke or a heart attack. (Atheroma is greek for porridge – a suitable description!) Blood pressure should be regularly monitored during pregnancy, as any sudden increase in blood pressure could lead to pre-eclampsia and complications for mother and baby. (See Pre-Eclampsia)

Calming, soothing and relaxing essential oils that have been shown to reduce hypertension include Lavender, Marjoram and Ylang Ylang. Reduction and elimination of animal fats, salt and alcohol, along with eating garlic, are all detoxifying and effective in normalising the pressure. If pregnant, use Neroli, Lavender and Rose, (Rose diluted to half normal strength), in a $2\frac{1}{2}$% dilution as a leg massage.

Hippocrates:
Hippocrates was a Greek physician, 460-370BC, known as the father of medicine. He had a great knowledge of plant medicines and holistic treatment, believed that we are a completely integrated system and that symptoms are as a result of a cause. He taught as he lived, by example, earning great love and respect. The Hippocratic Oath is taken today by doctors, to bind them to a moral code of ethics and practice, to protect life at all costs (sometimes Life more than the patient...).

Hives: (Also see Allergies)
Hives, also known as *Urticaria* or *Nettle Rash*, is an acute or

chronic allergic reaction in which lumps or weals, sometimes quite alarmingly large, appear on the skin. Common causes are strawberries or shellfish and the resulting rash can be infernally itchy and cause great discomfort. In children, hives can appear as though the child has been in a fight, but don't panic, check to see what they have been eating before you have a reaction yourself! They may last for an hour or so, or for a few days. If longer, then see your GP.

Use 3 drops of Chamomile and three of Melissa, to one cupful of carrier oil. Add one tablespoonful of the blend to a warm, not hot, bath – or gently paint on to the affected area with a wide, soft paintbrush.

Holistic:

Holistic treatment is treating the whole person, not a separate part or individual symptom, where the physical, mental and social factors are considered. Mind, body and spirit are accounted for, the cause or causes being of prime concern, not specifically the diagnosed disease or symptoms.

Homoeopathy:

The system of Homoeopathy was founded by Samuel Hahnemann, a German physician and chemist, at the end of the 18th century and is widely used today to treat all manner of disease and ailments. It is a system of medicine based on the principle of "like curing like". The patient is treated with infinitisimally small amounts of homoeopathic medication, which is capable of producing symptoms of his particular disease, thereby stimulating the body and its natural healing capacity to effect a cure.

As in aromatherapy, increased potency will not give increased benefit, less is more in both cases.

Hypertension: (See High Blood Pressure)

Hypoglaecemia:

When suffering from hypoglaecemia, the level of glucose in the bloodstream is too low. This deficiency can lead to muscular weakness, mental confusion, incoordination and sweating. It can commonly be caused by an inability to assimilate, or insufficient intake of, carbohydrates thus limiting their consequent conversion to glucose, or by insulin overdose. Treatment is to administer glucose, by mouth or by injection if the patient is in a coma. Robert Tisserand recommends the use of Eucalyptus to lower blood sugar levels, so this oil should be *avoided* if susceptible to Hypoglaecemia.

Hypotension: (See Low Blood Pressure)

Hypothalmus:
The hypothalmus is composed of a number of groups of nerve cells and is directly linked to the posterior and anterior lobes of the pituitary gland. The pituitary controls the release of hormones that are responsible for contracting the uterus around the time the baby is due, and to prime the muscles in preparations for contractions and labour.

The hypothalmus also exercises influence over the *autonomic nervous system*, which is in turn responsible for all the functions in our body over which we have no control. Hunger, thirst, heart beat, blood pressure, salivation and bodily secretions, intestinal movements etc., are all regulated by the ANS, along with the reflex nervous action, the involuntary reaction to stimulation to protect us from harm.

Immunity: (Immune System)
Immunity is the body's ability to resist infection, this ability being governed by the efficiency of our immune system. Those working with essential oils have a high resistance to illness. When the immune system is depleted, immune response requires stimulation, firstly by directly opposing invading organisms, and secondly, by strengthening activity of the organs and cells involved. Prolonged stress exhausts the adrenals, thus lowering the body's resistance to infection.

Following an attack of a disease, the body's cells produce appropriate antibodies to fight the invasion. Babies have a passive immune system for several weeks after birth, until their own immune systems are established. They are protected by antibodies - proteins that fight infection, and other types of protective proteins called immunoglobulins. Their immunity is passed on from the mother via maternal blood through the placenta and by *colostrum*. Innate immunity is present from birth. (See Breast Feeding) Allergies often begin before five years old, and are often as a result of an exaggerated immune response to a substance which is not necessarily harmful. The Thymus gland, behind the sternum, plays a vital part in the body's immunity by producing T-Lymphocytes to combat viral and other infections. It is small at birth (approx. 12g), and grows until puberty, when it begins to atrophy after reaching between 30 & 40g. By middle age it is back to the approximate weight at birth. In the child, the Thymus is very active, and like all lymphoid tissue, declines with age - so make the most of it!

From ages five to 12 the adaptive immune system is developing in complexity, with all the coughs, colds and other childhood infections encountered at this time, helping in this development. Children of all ages need a healthy diet and lifestyle to promote strong immunity, so encourage a prefer-ence (or even a liking!) for fresh foods, particularly fruit and vegetables. When a new infection is encountered, B-Lymphocytes produce antibodies to fight particular bacteria. Some of these cells remain as memory cells and recognise the return of the same bacteria and are ready to fight invasion at the first onset. This is known as Humoral Immunity and is of particular importance against bacterial infections. Cellular Immunity refers to the production of killer cells known as T-Lymphocytes, and are vital to protect us from invading viruses or tumours.

During the teenage years, immunity is usually strong, although a healthy diet is still essential. "Safe sex" is equally important as protection against HIV, the virus which can lead to AIDS (Aquired Immune Deficiency Syndrome), which dam-ages the crucial T-cells in the system and opens the door to infection.

From about 35 years old, although the immune system is still functioning, rheumatoid arthritis is common to begin now, affecting more women than men, so pay particular attention to a healthy lifestyle, both inside and out (See lymphatics). If healthy and your immune resistance is strong, you are less likely to be susceptible to degenerative and debilitating diseases and thus prevent premature ageing, so look after your immune system and help it care for you.

To help boost the immune system, massage with essential oils over and around the kidney area, in particular, where the adrenal glands that help to control the system lie.

To increase immune response and also act against a wide variety of bacteria, use either of the following in 50mls:

Bergamot	10 drops	or	Lavender	10 drops
Lavender	8 drops		Geranium	6 drops
Eucalyptus	4 drops		Tea Tree	6 drops
Tea Tree	4 drops		Rosemary/Black Pepper	3 drops

A healthy immunity also invloves a healthy lifestyle, and Aromatherapy can only help, not solve the problem. A balanced diet, with plenty of fresh foods, adequate exercise and nothing in excess, can establish a strong and healthy system able to deal with most infection.

Impetigo:
Impetigo is a highly contagious bacterial skin infection, especially virulent in communities of children, being easily spread by their regular physical contact and sharing of towels etc. Impetigo is not common in newborn babies today, however an outbreak may quickly spread in a maternity unit.

The infection is more commonly caused by *staphlococci*, although sometimes by *streptococci*. It begins as a red patch that rapidly spreads over the body forming yellow, crusty sores. Treatment must begin as soon as possible to prevent infection spreading, either to another person, or from one area to another on the same person. Conventional treatment involves the use of antibiotics, usually applied locally.

For a home treatment using aromatherapy, follow below:
Ensure the area is clean and as free from infected pus as possible. Clean the area with 15 drops of Lavender added to one litre of cooled, previously boiled water. Once thoroughly mixed, divide the mixture, leaving sufficient for a compress. After cleaning, leave the area exposed to the air for 10 minutes or so, to ensure it is as dry as possible, then apply

the compress to which you have added three drops of Tea Tree. Apply as often as possible, alternating with as much exposure to the air as possible, until the sores clear.

Impotence:
Unlike frigidity, impotence affects function in addition to enjoyment and fullfillment. (See Frigidity), and use oils of Patchouli, Sandalwood, Clary Sage and Ylang Ylang.

Massage the solar plexus (See Solar Plexus) in particular and use fragrance burners, light bulb rings or sprinkle a few drops of the favourite oil or oils around the room.

Indigestion:
Basil, Fennel, Chamomile, Lavender and Peppermint are effective against indigestion or dyspepsia, any combination of two of the above in a $2^1/2$% dilution rubbed on the stomach and sternum area of the chest should give substantial relief.

Unfortunately, when pregnant, the effective oils to combat indigestion or heartburn are the ones to be avoided, but Peppermint and Chamomile teas can help considerably. If indigestion really is a problem, do consult a professional aromatherapist for more specialist advice.

Avoid fatty, strongly flavoured or spicy foods, as these can cause increased acidity in the stomach. This is made even worse by over eating, or not eating regularly, worry or tension, often creating a vicious circle of stress, which of course makes the condition even worse. Try to relax, ensure you are breathing properly and that your posture is not cramping your insides. Extra pillows can help, as can milk at bedtime. Over-the-counter remedies that are safe and effective, include Remegel and Rapeze, especially if indigestion is accompanied by nausea, as they are both "non-chalky".

Infection:
As with all wounds and open skin, it is imperative to keep the area clean, free from infection and to promote healing. Lavender, Tea Tree and Chamomile essential oils are highly effective for all wounds. See the entry under accidents for further information.

Infertility:

It has been estimated that one in eight couples have problems conceiving. Identifying the problem and the need for factual and appropriate information is paramount, as is understanding, sympathy and commitment from those from whom help is sought.

It is a miracle to be able to make a baby at all, as so much is dependant on so many thousands of things. Sometimes, the deep sadness at being unable to have a family make the couple give up or adopt, and so often this is when conception finally takes place, once all the pressures have been eliminated. Apart from the sheer miracle of it all, a great deal depends on the mystery too, as sometimes there is no medical reason at all why a couple should not start a family. Stress, anxiety and how you feel emotionally, have a direct affect on chances of conception, added to the fact that there are only about 28 "really opportune" days each year, on which the average woman is able to conceive. The other 50% of possible complication could be related to the male, who before all else, has to have healthy sperm.

There are countless reasons why a couple may be unable to conceive, involving endless tests and medical examinations, all adding to the emotional stress which commonly prevents conception in the first place. Essential oils can certainly help with the emotional stress and tension, also by helping to harmonise the hormones involved in actual conception.

A shift in almost any hormone, sex related or otherwise, has an effect on mood and emotions. Psychological symptoms are often used to diagnose hormonal imbalance, emotional stress occuring most noticeably in women with varying hormonal levels, in particular before, during and after menstruation, pregnancy and birth. The Hypothalmus affects our emotions and influences our nervous system and the activities of many glands secreting hormones (See *Hypothalmus*). Aromatherapy can help to restore hormonal balance, including the feelings of being able to conquer the world one day, and being unable to order the milk the next. Keep a note in your diary of all the changes you feel, until a regular, and often suprising pattern emerges. This will help in establishing a suitable treatment from whichever or whatever professional and specialist body you choose to consult. Dr Jean Valnet refers to the phytohormonal properties of essential oils, in the way that certain plant hormones imitate our own. Decaux also drew attention to the fact that certain vegetable hormones contain sexual hormones.

There are many oils that can and do help, however establishing a correct balance of hormonal activity and treating possible hormonal insufficiency is essential. Consult a professional therapist.

Inflammation: (See Oedema)

Influenza:
'Flu is often blamed for any one of countless infections. However, as with all severe colds and viral infections, the treatment is virtually the same. It is vital for treatment to commence at the very first sign of the condition.

Rest, with as much sleep as possible, will help to support an immune system that has already been working very hard on your behalf before you even felt off colour. Once the infection begins to take hold, you need to do all you can to boost your immunity, helping the system to work at maximum efficiency and so restore good health as soon as possible. (See Immunity)
Use:
Tea Tree, Lavender and Eucalyptus in the bath, in the bedroom as a room vaporisor, but more effectively, in an inhalation. The main priority is to attack the invading virus and boost immunity.

Once recovery is on the way, include Bergamot in the treatment, especially in the bedroom, as this increases vitality, and Frankincense in the bath to fortify and rejuvenate. (Also see Colds and Fever)

Injuries: (See Accidents)

Insect Bites/Stings:
For any insect bites or stings, dab one drop of neat Lavender or Tea Tree to the area.

Insomnia:

For lack of sleep due to worries and anxieties, use Benzoin. For emotional distress use Neroli, Lavender or Chamomile. If the insomnia is due to over excitement, use Marjoram (but never if in a depressed state of mind), or Lavender.

Using the above essential oils in conjunction with a balanced diet, suitable exercise and relaxation techniques should break the vicious circle often created by lack of sleep and the accompanying distress it can cause. Place a few drops of the oils around the bed for children, and on the pillow, or on top of the duvet or sheet for adults. For babies and toddlers, avoid the bedroom as being a play area, keep it as a warm and relaxing place to be, with snuggly and cosy associations.

Bathe before bed, adding oils of your choice to a maximum of eight drops, and have as much massage as you can. Massage has been shown to consistently reduce stress and enhance relaxation, balance and well being. For babies and toddlers, up to five years old, dilute the oils first in a little carrier oil and mix thoroughly:

Lavender	2 drops
Roman Chamomile	1 drop
Melissa	1 drop

For those five years to 14, use:

Chamomile, either Roman or German	3 drops
Lavender	2 drops
Melissa	1 drop

Use the above equally effectively in a massage blend to the same proportions, ½% for toddlers, and 1% for five to 14 year olds.

Jealousy:

Some do and some don't know what this emotion feels like. For some it can be an emotion of rage, for others great heartbreak and sadness. Those who feel the emotion of jealousy need support and strengh to confront themselves and their insecurities, to hopefully avoid this damaging emotion. Oils to help, include Rose, Chamomile, Neroli, Sandalwood and Geranium.

Labour: (See Birth)

Laryngitis: (Also see Sore Throat and Tonsilitis)
Laryngitis can often make you lose voice. It is caused by infection or irritation and is inflammation of the larynx and vocal cords. Breathing can become difficult, often accompanied by a painful cough. An effective if somewhat painful remedy, is to "grab" and massage the sternocleidomastoid muscle on either side of the neck. This muscle serves to turn and rotate the head and is pronounced enough to "grab", if the head is turned fully to one side. Oils to use for laryngitis include:

Lavender   5 drops (2)
Chamomile   4 drops (2)
Tea Tree   4 drops (2)

Massage the above in 25mls, all around throat and chest area. Also inhale with steam as often as possible, as per the amounts in brackets.

Lice:
Lice are brownish grey in colour, and love the comfort of the scalp, where they find food and warmth. They lay six to eight eggs each day, which hatch after seven to 10 days. Their eggs are white in colour and are laid close to the skin, the empty shells being known as nits. Each louse takes two weeks to mature and if not detected, lives for 20 to 30 days. Nits and lice are very common, especially in children, and bear no relationship whatsoever to degrees of hygiene or cleanliness, they pass from head to head with the greatest of ease, the same louse could visit several heads in one day. They cannot jump or fly, they are passed on by close contact, so do inform friends or family, then elimination can be effective.

To check if your child has head lice, inspect the water after a hair wash, as lice and nits float. They also love the warm spots behind the ears, at the nape of the neck and under fringes, so check these areas regularly too. Lice quickly scuttle away should you part the hair to look for them, so are not so very easy to spot - the eggs or nits, are much easier to see. Ensure that hair is brushed and combed very thoroughly and regularly, as this injures the lice and makes them fall off and die.

Rosemary		Rose
Geranium		Geranium
Lavender	or	Lavender
Eucalyptus		Tea Tree
Lemon		

Both in equal parts to 100 mls of carrier oil (maximum 60 drops). Massage well into scalp and hair, wrap the head in cling film and leave for two hours. Work shampoo into the scalp and hair before adding water, this to break down the blend and enable the oils to be washed out. Apply the blend three times over 10 days, (every three days), leave for one week and repeat. Also add two drops each of Rosemary and Lavender, one drop of Eucalyptus to the rinse water after a normal hair wash, to help deter the "little creatures" in the first place.

Low Blood Pressure: (Hypotension)

Hypotension or low blood pressure is far less common than hypertension and also less serious. Symptoms include, frequent tiredness and dizzy spells. Regular exercise to increase efficient circulation and to get the blood pumping efficiently can help greatly, although take it slowly at first.

Use essential oils to stimulate and as a tonic, and massage as often as possible in gentle but firm movements to improve and stimulate circulation:

Rosemary	12 drops
Geranium	8 drops
Black Pepper	2 drops
Peppermint	2 drops - in 50mls.

Lungs:

The lungs and skin are the two main ways for essential oils to enter the blood stream. Essential oils are extremely volatile substances, the molecules in the air being inhaled through the nose and mouth. The exchange of gasses in the lungs, whereby oxygen and the goodies in essential oils are absorbed into the system, are exchanged with waste carbon dioxide. The molecules in the oils pass through the delicate thin walled capillaries in the lungs, and enter the blood stream to circulate and influence parts of the body. (See circulation)

Lymphatics:

The *Lymphatic* system, is made up of a network of vessels conveying lymph from tissue fluids to the bloodstream via *lymphatic vessels*. This extracellular fluid which bathes and nourishes the cells in the body, is purified by the lymphatic system.

Lymph nodes are groups of small swellings found at various points along the lymphatic system, such as in the armpit, behind the knee, in the elbows, in the groin and behind the ear. They produce *lymphocytes*, the white blood cells involved in establishing our immunity, and also act as filters for the lymph, filtering out and ensuring any waste products in the system cannot pass back into the blood and into circulation once more. When in the lymph vessels, the extracellular fluid is known as lymph. Although similar to plasma, it contains lymphocytes and less protein than plasma.

Massage and exercise play a major part in *lymphatic drainage,* helping to pump the lymph through the body, helping to strenthen the immune system and eliminate waste from the body. Unlike blood circulation, lymph is not pumped around the system by heart beat, its circulation is dependant on muscular contraction and relaxation, hence the value of massage and adequate exercise. The effect of increased levels of progesterone on smooth muscle during pregnancy, often leads to heartburn, constipation, indigestion and various aches and pains. Demand on the lymphatic system also increases. There are benefits too however, as the hormone helps the body to "soften" to accomodate baby and to ease delivery.

When the body is unhealthy, injured or under strain, the lymphatic system does not function efficiently, this often resulting in a build up of toxins and waste products and swellings usually at the sight of lymph nodes. Stimulation of the lymphatics with appropriate essential oils speeds up this elimination process.

Use:

Geranium	10 drops
Rosemary	8 drops
Patchouli	5 drops
Juniper	2 drops - in 30 mls, also in bath.

Massage is more specialist for lymph drainage, and should be extremely light, gently rhythmic and slow, this as the lymph vessels are very close to the surface of the skin. Always move towards the direction of the nearest lymph nodes, in particular the collar bone and the main area of drainage.

Massage:
A compassionate touch is comforting, firm and sensitive. With the action of touch begins all manner of communication and exchange. There are countless forms of body contact therapies, massage being a very primitive instinct and along with smell, touch is one of the first and most important senses to experience. From the early weeks of life, from conception to birth, the exploration of the texture, softness, temperature and odour of skin is a source of delight, wonder and learning, for all.

The language of skin contact is as difficult to describe and explain as the language of smell, but from this early handling and contact, comes our birth into adulthood and our ability to value touch, pleasure, experience and trust. Skin satisfaction is one of the most important infant experiences - the benefits of which should not be lost in adulthood, when some are not touched at all, either socially or sexually. Skin and muscle are not programmed to function separately and massage is a way through any blockages or insecurities that may be preventing that communication. Much response can be gained by massage with essential oils, to work on the physical, spiritual and emotional realms, to reach another by reading their reactions and gaining their trust. No two people are alike in their response to touch, massage or odour, all have different needs, wants and wishes, so during a massage, let your own intuitions and those of the one you are massaging, run freely, with sensitivity and care.

There are numerous books on the cumulative benefits and countless forms of massage, but massage using essential oils is the most influential application of aromatherapy.

For various recipies see relevant entry.

For a general baby massage formula, for three - 12months:

Roman Chamomile	1 drop
Lavender	1 drop
Geranium	1 drop, diluted in 30 mls of carrier.

Mastitis: (Also see Abscess/Breasts)

Mastitis is inflammation of the breast, usually as a result of bacterial infection via the nipples, commonly occuring during breast feeding.

Chronic cystic mastitis is a different condition, thought to be caused by hormone imbalance, and does not normally cause inflammation. Breasts feel "lumpy" and painful. As with all conditions concerning the breasts, if not quickly remedied, check up with your GP.

Measles:

Never dismiss measles, even though the virus has virtually been eradicated, it can be a killer. Measles are highly contagious, children being especially vulnerable to any bacterial infection at the early stages of the virus. The first sign is an outbreak of spots in the mouth, spreading to the cheeks and chest as a rash. The virus is spread by saliva and by airborne bacteria. Use room vaporisers or sprays. (See *Rubella* and *Rashes*)

Menstruation:

Premenstrual Tension, or Premenstrual Syndrome, correlates with low levels of oestrogen and high progesterone, just before a period. This can have a profound effect upon the emotions. Symptoms include swollen and tender abdomen and breasts, poor skin quality and spots, depression, crying and irritability - to fluid retention, headaches and nausea. When these levels balance out, mood, emotions and physical symptoms dramatically improve. Before giving birth, oestrogen levels are up about 1000 over the previous level - after birth, this level plummets, the reaction being a common cause of post-natal depression.

If for you, "irregular periods" is the norm, and you experience no difficulties, then apart from not really knowing where you are, and having to "be prepared" just in case, there is no problem. Only when bleeding suddenly becomes irregular should you require investigation to ensure all is well to prevent possible complication.

An *endometrial biopsy* may be done to check the condition of the endometrial lining of the uterus. There could be complication due to fibroids, polyps, or it might even be a hormone problem. Any shift in hormone levels, for whatever reason, can have a profound effect. Emotional stress is the most common cause of varying hormone levels, especially during pregnancy and after. Don't ever take chances if there is a sudden change from your normal pattern. The cause is more than likely something easily remedied, but cancer is a remote possibility too, so please don't risk it.

Amenorrhoea, is the absence or stopping of menstruation. An *emmenagogue* induces menstruation. These oils include Basil, Clary Sage, Fennel, Juniper, Marjoram, Myrrh, Peppermint, Rose and Rosemary. For obvious reasons, these oils must be avoided during pregnancy. Lavender and Chamomile have been classed as mild emmenagogues, however, unless there is a risk of miscarriage, these oils are generally safe to use after the first trimester, in normal doses, but if in any doubt, consult a professional aromatherapist.

Menorrhagia, or excessive blood loss, is often associated with hormonal imbalance and is common to those suffering from PMS, therefore avoid the above oils if this applies.

Approximately half of all pre-menopausal women who menstruate, suffer from PMT/PMS. Women whose health and immunity is good, tend to suffer less than those who suffer ill health and from lack of exercise and good nutrition. The body eliminates waste by many means, including menstruation, which can often be the cause of heavy bleeding, cramps and spasms in the womb and associated areas. The fatigue and fluid retention, commonly associated with PMS, is due to the extra strain on the adrenal and thyroid glands, liver and kidneys during this detoxifying process, thus resulting in the heaviness in the pelvic region, and often those tell-tale spots and acne appearing, as waste is eliminated through the skin. A good diet is essential, especially during the week to 10 days before a period is due - including as much fresh and raw food as possible, such as salads, vegetables, fruit, water and natural juices, this to aid the elimination process. Avoid simple carbohydrates, such as white bread and flour, refined sugary drinks and foods, chocolate and sweets, and stick to complex carbohydrates including wholemeal bread, pasta, potatoes, brown rice and pulses. These are more slowly absorbed into the system and help to maintain a constant blood sugar level. The common and often severe hunger cravings frequently experienced in the few days before a period, is believed by many specialists to be as a result of a drastic fall in blood sugar, or Hypoglycaemia (see entry). This produces a rush of the hormone adrenaline into the system - often leading to panic attacks, migraine, mood swings and temper. Also avoid salt, tea, coffee, alcohol, and restrict dairy products as much as possible, as they are mucous forming. Foods rich in iron to help replace loss during blood flow can also help considerably, along with vitamin C to help aid absorption, vitamin A and B complex, and Evening Primrose Oil, being rich in GLA. (See Evening Primrose Oil)

Here's Health, January 1989, Leon Chaitow/November 1990, Dr Mike Whiteside.

For general symptoms of PMT/PMS:

Clary Sage	10 drops
Geranium	10 drops
Rose	3 drops

Massage over the whole body, in 25mls of carrier oil. For self help, massage over lower back, solar plexus, tops of thighs and buttocks and over abdomen. Do this approximately one week before "the curse" is due, and for approximately one week afterwards. Unless the condition improves quickly, continue for several periods. (Also see Oedema)

For irregular or absent periods:

Basil	2 drops
Fennel	2 drops
Melissa/Rose	2 drops – as a compress.

For painful periods use:

Clary Sage	15 drops
Chamomile	5 drops
Geranium	5 drops
Rose	2 drops

Miscarriage: (Also see Abortion and Grief)

More than half of all pregnancies end in miscarriage, some known about, some not. In many cases, the woman is not even aware that she has conceived and that the fertilized egg has not implanted in the uterus, before her next normal period. Some miscarriages occur slightly later, as a delayed or heavier than normal period, and some 15% of recognisable miscarriages happen later still. If this occurs during the first 10 weeks of pregnancy, this is normally due to abnormal development of the embryo, and is nature's way of taking care of its own mistake.

Unless you have a history of miscarriage, normal rest, relaxation and caring for yourself and your baby, and avoiding unnecessary risk is the norm. Being pregnant does not mean you are ill, and horrific stories of females drinking bottles of gin, having scalding hot baths and hurling themselves downstairs, has often done nothing to dislodge a healthy, but unwanted baby, except perhaps untold harm to the mother and possibly the child. However, bleeding during pregnancy can be a sign that you are overdoing things and should rest, or if accompanied by severe cramps and clots, miscarriage is usually inevitable. Bleeding does not necessarily mean you are going to lose the baby however, often bed rest and relaxation is all that is needed. Listen to your body.

For many women, the emotional consequences of losing a baby by miscarriage can be great. For some, hopes and dreams of many years might have been depending on the lost baby, and any hopes of happiness disappear. Miscarrying can be seen as punishment, as their own fault and many suffer great feelings of guilt and depression. Whatever the reason, and however emotions are felt, the quickest way back to recovery is a must, both physically and emotionally. Waiting at least three months, or for three menstrual cycles is known to reduce the statistical risk of miscarrying again - the longer the better. However, waiting three months, would mean the due date would co-incide with the lost baby's birthday. You need to feel able to start afresh, and the following pregnancy should not be an extension of the last. If you expect to use the same hospital for your successful pregnancy a pre-pregnancy visit to "lay any ghosts" may be helpful. It is obviously natural that once a woman has miscarried, she should be anxious about a recurrence during any following pregnancy. This is not necessarily so, although the chances are increased very slightly.

Use Geranium, Roman Chamomile, Rose, Frankincense, Neroli, Grapefruit, Orange.

For emotional and spiritual healing:

Frankincense	9 drops
Geranium	9 drops
Benzoin/Bergamot	7 drops
Neroli	4 drops - in 50mls.

(Also see Abortion and Grief)

Morning Sickness: (See Nausea)

Mouth Ulcers:
Use a cotton bud with one drop of essential oil of Tea Tree if pregnant or Myrrh if not, and dab directly on to ulcer. Repeat as necessary.

Mumps:
Mumps is a contagious viral disease, symptoms showing as swellings of the parotid glands on either side of the face and below the ears, this due to inflammation of the salivary glands. Other glands can sometimes be affected, this occasionally including the testicles and pancreas. The incubation period for mumps is 2 - 4 weeks.

The oils to use for home use are Tea Tree, Lavender, and Lemon or Grapefruit - in equal parts in the bath (max 10 drops), in a diffuser, vaporiser, or preferably as an inhalation (max. two drops of each). Dosage should be three times each day, for maximum of 10 days. Take lots of rest and drink much water and fruit juice. For more specialist treatment consult a professional aromatherapist.

Muscles: (Also see Massage)
To stimulate circulation, and relieve aches and pains, cramps and muscle fatigue, massage is the most effective remedy. Use:

Lavender	12 drops
Rosemary/Lemongrass	7 drops
Juniper	6 drops

or

Rosemary/Lemongrass	10 drops
Geranium	8 drops
Black Pepper	2 drops

Use in 30mls of oil, also in bath.

During pregnancy use:

Sandalwood	8 drops
Orange/Petitgrain	8 drops
Frankincense	8 drops

In 50mls of oil.

Nails:

The condition of the body shows in the nail. When under certain medical supervision, nail varnish is removed to permit monitering of the body's condition. Care of the cuticle bed is most important, as any damage or infection can seriously affect the whole nail. Essential oils make the nails grow fast and furiously, which is fine if you enjoy long, luxurious and very strong nails, but when in a busy practice, nails have to be short and manageable, and have to be cut almost every other day.

To strengthen nails:

Lemon	3 drops	Lemongrass	3 drops
Rosemary	2 drops	Lavender	2 drops

For a cuticle softener:

Eucalyptus	3 drops
Peppermint	2 drops

For infection in or around the nail bed:

Tea Tree	3 drops
Lavender	2 drops
Lemon/Patchouli	1 drop

For all the above, pour a little amount of Almond oil into the palm of your hand and mix the essential oils in well, or add the drops to a desertspoonful of oil in an egg cup or something similar. Only a little amount is needed. Massage into the cuticle and nail area daily.

Nappy Rash:

Nappy rash is normally caused by the delicate skin being warm, wet and airless, the air being unable to circulate around sodden skin which quickly becomes sore. Once urine or faeces comes into contact with the skin in this condition, it is much more likely to sting and cause a rash. Gradually her skin becomes tougher the older baby gets, but dampness can still cause problems.

Frequent nappy changes are a must, especially as a new born baby urinates every 20–30 minutes on average! Some commercial wet-wipes and disposable nappies in combination, can cause reaction, as can scented nappy liners. The use of water washing and thorough drying is the cheapest method, and by far the best. Before baby is more active, and sleeps a lot of the time, as long as she is warm enough, allow her to sleep on a nappy, rather than in one, letting the air dry her skin. She will probably love the freedom.

Protective/barrier creams also prevent the air as well as moisture reaching the skin, so avoid using them when she is open to the air, but use more at night to protect a sore bottom. Avoid over creaming the inner folds of the groin and although vaseline helps prevent meconium (newborn's first stools), from adhering to the skin in the first few days of life, avoid use after stools have changed colour.

If nappy rash does develop, and it possibly will, no matter how careful you are, prevent it developing further by acting quickly. It can start with slight redness and heat, quickly progressing to inflammation, with sores and eventually yellow pustules, causing considerable distress both to you and baby. The acid from urine stings moist, sore skin, the bacteria from stools or unsterilised nappies then causing infection.

The area should be kept clean and as dry as possible. Let as much air as you can get to the area, allowing the older child to play in the sunshine if practical, with adequate sun-block protection, and allow her the freedom of being naked with the air on her skin.

Into approximately one litre of cooled, previously boiled water, add Chamomile and Lavender, one drop of each. Rinse the area and dry thoroughly. Add one drop of each oil to a dessertspoonful of barrier cream such as zinc and castor oil (no lanolin), or sudocrem, and cover the area. Repeat at each change until the area is clear again.

Nausea:
Feeling nauseous and actually vomiting is a natural reaction - if it's felt, let it happen. Recurrent vomiting is unnatural however, and should be investigated. Listen to your body, as sometimes a dry biscuit or a drink might be the thing to settle the feeling, or the one thing to induce vomiting. If pregnant, drink Peppermint or Chamomile tea and keep a supply of dry biscuits available.

Some babies and children suffer projectile vomiting, whereby they are capable of projecting their vomit with such force as to travel several feet. This is normally due to a medical condition and should be investigated.

Peppermint oil calms the stomach and aids digestion, also helping with the disorientation often associated with nausea. Place a drop on a handkerchief and inhale when necessary. Also use Lavender or Fennel.

In addition to inhaling the above oils, use a compress with two drops of oil added to one litre of water. Inhalation or a compress is preferably to use when feeling nauseous, as massage can make the condition worse. Place the compress over the forehead, holding it there as a comfort often being an effective remedy.

Nerves/Nervous System:
Our *neurological system* has two main divisions, the *central nervous system*, and the *autonomic nervous system*, at the centre of which is the brain. The spinal column of vertabrae protects the precious spinal cord, the continuation of the medulla oblongata region of the brain, and our nervous system. The nervous system is the most complex system of the body, being vital to our whole function, containing millions of supporting blood vessels, cells and nerves. Massage with essential oils along this area has maximum benefit, either sedative, stimulating or regulating.

The millions of nerves in the body, that collect and relay

information to and from the brain, travel via the spinal cord. They include *receptors* which respond to different stimuli, and those that carry the messages for reaction to the muscles and glands, known as *motor* nerves.

Reflex nervous action is an involuntary reaction to stimulation, often initiated by the spinal cord instead of the brain, usually in cases of necessary immediate action to prevent harm. In a case of handling a hot plate for example, the reflex action of dropping the plate immediately, before the pain message has reached the brain, is initiated by the spinal cord. If however, the reflex action is initiated by the brain, the pain message having time to get there (we are talking less than split seconds here!) the plate is quickly put down, thus preventing a broken plate, a lost dinner and more work. Our system is also conditioned by other considerations, such as intelligence and experience.

The autonomic nervous system is divided into two, the *Sympathetic*, which tends to stimulate body activity, and the *Parasympathetic*, which tends to slow down and regulate. Both are linked to the spinal cord from which they supply the necessary regions and organs. The sympathetic runs either side of the front of the spinal column and supplies the thoracic area, all the abdominal viscera and the pelvic organs. It is stimulated by strong emotions, such as anger or excitement, the adrenals releasing adrenalin in response to anger for example. Those who tend to be more emotional are usually dominated by stronger sympathetic nerves, those dominated by the parasympathetic holding the balance, are generally more placid and not easily disturbed.

To calm and soothe:

Chamomile	10 drops
Lavender	8 drops
Rose	8 drops

When pregnant:

Melissa	10 drops
Rosewood	5 drops
Orange/Neroli	3 drops

Neuralgia: (Also see Sciatica)

Neuralgia is pain originating in a nerve. Sciatica is a a common form of neuralgia, the Sciatic nerve being the longest in the body. Analgesic essential oils include Chamomile, Peppermint, (maximum two drops), Lavender, Clary Sage, Marjoram and Rosemary. A combination of any two to three oils on a warm compress should be used on the affected area or areas. Place a hot water bottle on top if necessary, and relax as much as possible.

Nits: (See Lice)

Nose Bleeds:

Nose bleeds are common in children and also in pregnancy. Usually they right themselves in time and are the body's natural way of releasing pressure. Place a cold compress, if you feel it necessary, over the bridge of the nose, and pinch the nose immediately below the bone of the bridge, maintaining even pressure until bleeding stops.

Haemostatic essential oils speed up the rate of blood clotting and include Geranium and Rose, however with nose bleeds, I would recommend the natural process taking its course.

Oedema: (Also see Cellulite and Menstruation)

Oedema is the resulting swelling due to excessive accumulation of fluid in the body tissues. It may be localised due to a sprain or injury and so only temporary, or generalised and due to a more serious condition such as kidney malfunction or a heart condition. *Subcutaneous oedema* commonly occurs in the fingers, wrists, legs and ankles, due to the level of gravity, and is common during pregnancy and before menstruation. It can also occur facially and in the sacral and abdominal wall. Swelling can be greatly helped by rest and elevation of the legs and arms by lying down as much as possible. Subcutaneous, and localised oedema should cause no concern unless accompanied by high blood pressure, which can quickly lead to more serious complications, particularly during pregnancy when both mother and baby can be seriously affected. (See *pre-eclampsia*)

Fluid retention can also be associated with an allergy, or with an accumulation of waste in the body (see *lymphatic drainage*). The body has an effective, (if sometimes unsightly) way of rendering waste products less dangerous, by diluting them and minimising the harmful affects.

Effective detoxifying essential oils include Rosemary, Fennel, Grapefruit, Juniper and Lemon. Oils to help reduce fluid retention, especially pre-menstrually, include Geranium, Clary Sage, Rosemary and Fennel.

For puffiness associated with PMT:

Geranium	12 drops
Fennel	6 drops
Rosemary	5 drops
Clary Sage	5 drops

Use in 50mls of carrier oil and massage full body, or particularly around abdomen, legs and arms in long, smooth, firm strokes towards the heart. Begin one week before menstruation begins. This treatment also benefits the lymphatic system in draining excess fluids from the tissues.

For general detoxification:

Lemon	8 drops
Juniper	8 drops
Fennel	8 drops

Osteopathy:

Osteopathy is a system of healing based on joint manipulation concerning disorders of the musculoskeletal system. At the end of the 19th century, an American named Andrew Taylor Still discovered a cure for certain disorders by manipulation and correction of misaligned structure. Specific manipulation, of the spine in particular, affects joints, ligaments, muscles and associated organs and tissues.

Osteopathy works well in conjunction with holistic aromatherapy as it is concerned with treatment of the patient as a whole, not just the disorder - restoring balance physically, mentally and spiritually.

Many disorders respond well to osteopathy, in particular back pain and associated tensions and disease due to imbalance of structure and function Once a full consultation has taken place, the manipulative treatment involved may be very gentle or very firm, this depending on the patient's needs and constitution. Osteopaths have a high degree of sensitivity in their fingers and are trained in a method of examination known as palpation. This enables them to detect subtle changes in body tissue, muscles, ligaments tendons and joints etc.

Aromatherapy massage is of particular benefit in osteopathic treatment, relaxing and de-stressing the system either before, during or after a treatment, many osteopaths involving aromatherapy and aromatherapists in their work.

Otitis: (See Ear Ache)

Pain:
Pain is relative, a natural warning of danger to the system. Any prolonged pain in the same area should be investigated to prevent further complication arising. If in any doubt whatsoever, seek professional medical advice.

Pain relievers should be avoided if at all possible, especially in babies and young children, as they may mask something that needs treatment. If your child is in pain see your doctor. Essential oils stimulate the body's own natural pain killers, such as *endorphins*, (see entry) and *encephalins*.

Palpitations:
Normal increase and awareness of heart beat is a natural reaction to exertion, emotion or fear and palpitations are commonly felt during pregnancy. However, prolonged palpitations may be a symptom of a more serious condition concerning the heart or circulation and could be confused with *tachycardia*. Any increase in the heart beat above normal should be checked.

Comforting and calming essential oils include Neroli, Lavender, Chamomile and Ylang Ylang or Rose.

Perineal Massage: (Also see Episiotomy)
Massage of the perineum has been practised in different cultures throughout history. It is done ante-natally by the

mother or her partner during the last weeks of pregnancy, to make the perineum more supple and elastic to prepare the birth outlet and ease delivery, thus hopefully avoiding the need for an episiotomy.

Relaxation of the muscles before massage is helped by a warm aromatic bath to soften tissues and increase circulation, with oils of Geranium and Lavender added, four drops of each. Empty your bladder before beginning, and ensure you are comfortable and well supported. Make up a blend of two drops of Lavender to one drop of Geranium, in a 2½% dilution of almond oil.

Lubricate your two index fingers, or your thumbs, and the perineal area. Insert your fingers 3–4cms inside the vagina and press the perineal floor towards the rectum and to the sides in a "U" shape. If the clitoris is at 12 o'clock, then work between four and eight o'clock, paying particular attention to scar tissue from any previous episiotomy which will not stretch so easily. Maintain gentle stretch and pressure for approximately one minute, until you feel slight burning or tingling and the area becomes somewhat numb. After a few weeks the area will become noticeably more supple and the feelings associated with baby's head crowning will become more familiar. This area is particularly private and sensitive and once used to the feeling of stretch, the mother is less likely to respond with tension when it really is baby's head crowning. At this stage of birth, it is essential to be as relaxed as is possible to enable your baby to be born with your perineum intact. Pelvic floor exercises (the "lift going up to the penthouse and down to the basement...") after the birth, will soon tone up the stretched muscles.

If there is a history of herpes or any other infection during the pregnancy, avoid perineal massage due to possible spread of infection.

Periods: (See Menstruation)

Pets:
Pregnancy, babies, children and pets can and do go together very well, providing certain precautions are taken. (See

Toxoplasmosis). Apart from the obvious extra care in maintaining hygiene, and ensuring no harm can come to babies or children (or your pets!) being in the midst of family life and learning the caring and sharing can be a bonus for everybody, especially baby.

Most animals keep themselves clean, but some do not. Particular care should be taken in keeping pet food dishes and utensils out of reach and separate from family dishes, but keeping your child away from pet excreta is a must, either in your garden or in any public place. Serious disease can result from contact with bacteria from pet excreta, babies and pregnant women being the most at risk.

Once baby has understood that the family pets are not toys to be pulled at, poked and prodded, that they actually are part of the family and enjoy love and kindness too - and the animals have got over the trauma! - they will probably be the very best of friends. Never leave baby alone with animals, as no matter how loving and gentle your pets are, baby is very vulnerable, dogs may be jealous or want to "play", and cats love to snuggle over warm things. Whenever baby is asleep outside, always use a cat net for protection, and use it even when baby is taken out of the pram to keep out bugs, flies and wasps in particular.

Animals love being pampered, just as we humans do, and pampering is therapeutic for all concerned. My animals love a massage, and the cats have seriously been into reflexology for years!

For fleas, tics etc:

Tea Tree	4 drops
Eucalyptus	4 drops
Bergamot/Lemon	4 drops

Mix well in one litre of warm water and comb through the coat, avoiding the eye area. Repeat every other day for one week (three times). Repeat two weeks later.

For wounds:

Bathe in dilution of cup of cooled boiled water to which you have added three drops of Tea Tree and three drops of Lavender.

Piles: (See Haemorrhoids)

Placenta:
Full of hormones and nutrients, in some cultures the placenta is eaten raw by the mother, to restore health and vitality dramatically reduced after the birth. (See *birth*.) Animals eat it for nourishment as they are weakened after the birth and unable to hunt. Thank goodness for tea and toast!

P.M.T.: (See Menstruation)

Post Natal Peroid:
    After giving birth to your baby, you have effectively given your body and soul and just about everything there is, to bring her safely into this world. The energy output from you has been immense, and that energy and giving needs to be replenished. To be loved and feel loving is possibly the most valuable thing right now, and a massage or a bath with one of the following blends should work wonders.

Neroli/Orange	10 drops
Frankinsence	8 drops
Grapefruit	4 drops
Bergamot	10 drops
Clary Sage	8 drops
Rose	4 drops
Geranium	10 drops
Frankinsence	8 drops
Jasmine	4 drops

    Bedroom based rest for the first few days is recommended, with visiting restricted to those really close to you. Friends, be they relatives or not, are those that bring food, do the shopping or even the washing – not those who just want to cuddle the baby (usually when she is asleep), stay for hours and drink your tea and eat your fruit and leave you with the washing up! If that is the case – ask them to return at 4am when you will be thrilled with their help. (See Babymoon/Birth/Menstruation)

Posture: (See Back)

Pre-eclampsia
At your regular ante natal appointments, your blood pressure should be checked, your urine tested for the presence of protein and any signs of sudden or excessive fluid retention be noted. Any or all of these could be a sign of pre-eclampsia (pregnancy-induced hypertension).

The cause of this hypertension is as yet unknown, but is most commonly found in the first pregnancy of a union. Subsequent pregnancies are usually unaffected within the same partnership.

Regular ante-natal checks are essential as the best preventative measure of the condition progressing to *Eclampsia*, which must be treated immediately, as it is a serious threat to both mother and baby.

**Pyorrhoea – Gum inflammation/infection:
(See Gingivitis)**

Rashes:
A rash is classed as a temporary skin eruption, first shown as reddening, often with small red spots that itch. A rash can be a localised reaction to an external substance or an indication of an internal imbalance.

Rashes are very common in children and can appear as quickly as they disappear, often with no cause for concern. They can also be associated with infectious diseases such as measles however, so as usual, be safe rather than sorry and have it checked by a GP if uncertain.

Use Lavender   4 drops
Chamomile   4 drops

Add the essential oil to a warm, not hot bath, or halve the quantity and add to one litre of cool water or Chamomile tea and bathe the affected area. Alternatively paint the area with the blend, using a wide, soft paintbrush.

Reflexology:
Relexology, or *Zone Therapy*, is an effective system of diagnosis

and treatment of the whole system by working on the soles of the feet, the main theory being that every part of the body has a representative area on the foot. As in acupuncture, reflexology is based on treatment to unblock congestion in energy lines. These channels on the feet mirror the whole system and massage and pressure on these blockages releases congestion, thereby allowing energy to run freely once more, toning and harmonising the entire system and restoring health and well being.

Reflexology is an holistic treatment, that works especially well with aromatherapy. Certain imbalances that have been established can be treated by massage with appropriate essential oils, combined with reflexology to stimulate reflexes in the feet and help correct and maintain health in all parts of the body.

Rescue Remedy: (See Bach Flower Remedies)

Rhesus Disease:
Approximately 15% of women have blood classed as *Rhesus negative* and when a child is conceived by a father with *Rhesus positive* blood, the baby's blood may not match that of her mother's. In these cases, during labour when there is added pressure on the placenta, some of thebaby's blood may be squeezed back into the mother's system, the mother's cells then forming antibodies to deal with the invasion.

This can cause no problem to a first baby. However, for a second baby with a differing blood group, there may be a problem. The mother's blood, passing through the placenta to nourish her baby, may begin to attack the baby's blood cells, being different to her own, this leading to anaemia and jaundice as the baby's liver has to cope with eliminating the killed off cells. In the past, this condition frequently caused death to the baby whilst in the womb, but now can be prevented by careful monitoring after the first birth to ensure none of the *rhesus positive* blood cells have entered her circulation. If so, she is injected with rhesus positive cells to neutralise the foreign blood cells from her baby and thus prevent her making any further antibodies of her own.

Rheumatic Fever:

Rheumatic fever is a disease that mainly affects young adults and children. The main symptoms are fever, red patches on the skin and arthritis progressing from joint to joint, inflammation of the heart and small nodules forming on bony areas such as the elbow. Conventional treatment is to treat initial symptoms with antibiotics and much healing rest, however an acute attack can lead to much more long term treatment. Always seek professional advice.

Ringworm:

Ringworm is a form of fungi affecting the outer layer of skin. Athletes foot is a form of ringworm, also being highly contagious and infernally itchy. As its name suggests, the infection is ringlike.

Apply one drop of Tea Tree, neat on the area, morning and evening, for one week. Leave for one week and apply daily for a second week.

Also use Lavender five drops and Tea Tree five drops, in the bath. As an alternative, use 30 drops in 30mls of oil, 15 of each, to cover the larger surrounding area.

Rubefacient:

Any area that requires warmth and stimulation can benefit from a rubefacient essential oil. These include Black Pepper, Peppermint, Eucalyptus, Juniper, Marjoram and Rosemary. These oils stimulate the area and increase circulation, often causing redness. Because these oils are so stimulating, only a low amount is required.

Rubella:

Rubella, or German Measles, although not as serious as measles, can cause fetal abnormality if contracted within the first four months of pregnancy. Women planning on becoming pregnant should check with their GP to ensure they are immune. Although the majority of children are vaccinated against Rubella, immunity can diminish, some people rejecting immunity from vaccination altogether.

Use room sprays and diffusers with anti-viral oils such as,

Lavender, Tea Tree, Eucalyptus and Rosemary, blended with Chamomile, Geranium or Lemon/Lemongrass. (Also see Rashes)

Safety: (See Accidents and Contra-indications/Toxicity/Dosage)

Scarlet Fever:
Scarlet fever is a *streptococcal* and highly contagious disease, the symptoms being a sore throat, fever and sickness. On day two or three, a rash appears on the chest and neck, often spreading to the whole body. The rash usually fades after approximately one week, when the skin can be dry and flake.

Possible complications of scarlet fever can include a middle ear infection and possible kidney infection. See your GP.

Treat as for *Tonsilitis* and *Rubella*, and use Lavender and Chamomile, three drops of each in a warm bath, or in a blend of six drops of Lavender with four drops of Chamomile in 25mls of oil.

Scarring:
Use Lavender, Bergamot, Chamomile, Frankincense or Neroli. Blend two or three oils together, preferably using Neroli with another, either in a cream or in a carrier such as wheatgerm oil. Apply daily to the scar for a minimum of eight weeks or until improvement.

Sciatica: (Also see Neuralgia)
This can refer to any pain along the *Sciatic Nerve*, the longest nerve in the body. As usual in any form of holistic treatment, the aim is to find and treat the cause, not just the symptom. Sciatica can cause quite distressing pain and a visit to the osteopath might be the answer, to check posture and any misalignment causing possible pressure or irritation along the nerve.

The sciatic nerve leaves the pelvis and the spine, passes below the sacroiliac joint to the buttocks, goes behind the hip joint, down the thigh and divides at the knee going down the calf to the foot. That gives much length and possibility for pain, from many possible causes, so check it out with a professional if it gives you regular trouble. It could of course be due to tiredness, bad posture or even sleeping or sitting in a bad position, so try some self help first. Irritation of the sciatic nerve is very common during pregnancy and is often due to increased pressure from the baby. Various aches and pains are often due to the pelvic structures softening in preparation for birth, so look on the positive side too!! Once baby is born, the problem usually disappears, but do seek out obstetric physiotherapy via your midwife or GP if the problem causes distress. Pelvic tilting exercises can be of great benefit along with the following.

Cold compresses over the area of pain can bring welcome relief, as can warm, relaxing baths, with oils of Lavender or Chamomile.

Sebum:
Sebum is one of the most valuable secretions from our body, being produced by the sebaceous glands which open up into the hair follicles and is the medium through which the essential oils enter our systems. There is only usually any complication or problem, when the secretion levels are out of balance. Sebum keeps the skin supple and protects it from outside influence, including unfriendly bacteria - too little, and skin becomes dehydrated and sensitive to outside influence - too much and pores become blocked and possibly infected.

For an excess of sebum, leading to over oily skin, use: Bergamot, Lemon, Juniper, and Cedarwood oils.

For too little, leading to dehydrated and sensitive skin, use: Neroli, Jasmine, Lavender, Rose and Chamomile.

Use either combination in a light, nutritious base oil of your choice, suitable for your skin, such as Peach Kernel or Almond with 10% of Wheatgerm, Jojoba or Avocado. (Also see Ageing)

Sensitivity: (See Toxicity and Contra-indications)

Shingles:
Shingles, or *Herpes Zoster*, also causes Chickenpox in children. The first symptom is pain in the face, chest or abdomen,

developing in tiny blisters similar to those occuring in eczema. The virus can lay dormant from childhood and flare up again in adulthood, commonly in conditions of stress when immunity is low. The condition can be very painful and distressing, as it affects the sensory nerves, the rash appearing on the areas of skin served by the affected nerves.

Use a combination of analgesic oils to ease pain, along with oils to treat the blisters and the accompanying distress. Try Bergamot and either Eucalyptus or Tea Tree, with Lavender and Chamomile.

Bergamot   10 drops
Lavender   8 drops
Eucalyptus   5 drops

Use in a 2½% dilution, gently smoothing the blend along the affected areas, in addition to all along the spinal area. Also add 10 drops of the blended mixture to the bath.

Shock:
Shock is a condition associated with circulatory collapse, when many vital functions are slowed down, sometimes seriously, owing to insufficient blood flow. The prevention and treatment of shock and its consequences, are of prime importance.

Although some degree of shock is expected, and very normal, in any case of accident or emergency, it is important to know how to combat the condition. Symptoms can include weakness, drop in temperature, perspiration, nausea, a rapid weak pulse and irregular breathing.

The most effective treatment for minor or emotional shock is *Rescue Remedy*. (See *Bach Flower Remedies*) although a direct sniff of Neroli or Lavender can also help.

For severe shock or collapse take the following course of action:

1 Keep the patient warm and still

2 Ensure all airways are unrestricted and clear

3 Any restrictive clothing should be loosened to ease circulation.

4 Stay as calm and reassuring as you can and get medical aid fast.

Sinus:

The sinuses are above, behind and at each side of the nose. They are air cavities within bone, lined with mucous membrane and are linked to the nasal cavities by small openings, easily blocked during any infection or increase in nasal mucous. When infection is trapped within the sinus, the passages being blocked by mucous, the resulting pain can be almost unbearable, often leading to sickness and temperature.

The most important treatment is to combat infection and to clear blocked passages.

Use inhalations of:

Eucalyptus	2 drops
Tea Tree	2 drops
Lavender	2 drops - 3 times per day.

Light massage of the area can help to drain congestion and ease pressure.

Use the following in light, gentle massage around the nose forehead, cheeks, ears and neck - in three tablespoons of oil:

Rosemary	2 drops
Geranium	2 drops
Chamomile	2 drops
Eucalyptus	1 drop

Acupuncture is also a very effective treatment for sinusitis. Make an appointment with a professional therapist if the condition is not quickly eased by self help treatment. Avoid all dairy produce as this is mucous forming.

Skin Care: (Also see Ageing, Thread veins, Acne and Sebum)

Problem skin is nearly always due to a sensitivity or an imbalance of sebum production. Fortunately, skin responds extremely well to aromatherapy, as the essential oils have direct benefits on tone, texture and oil balance. The skin on the face changes very rapidly, so bear this in mind when mixing your appropriate blends, changing them frequently for maximum benefit.

For baby, when dry and flaky in the little folds of indescribably soft and delicate skin, use the following:

| German Chamomile | 4 drops |
| Lavender | 2 drops |

Dilute well in 50 mls.

Smoking:

It is a known and established fact that smoking can cause heart disease, lung cancer and other diseases and thatabout one in every four smokers dies as a direct result of smoking. Many others suffer years of pain and discomfort. The only way to avoid being one of these statistics is to stop smoking, for you, those that love you, and, especially when pregnant, for your unborn child for whom you are directly responsible.

It could be one of the hardest things you do, especially if the circumstances of your pregnancy are particularly stressful or unhappy, but it is probably one of the most important things you can do. If you cannot do it on your own, get some help, and take it one day at a time. You will be giving up smoking for the very best reason that there is. Life.

For advice and details, contact:

Quit
Latimer House
40-48 Hanson Street
London W1P 7DE

Solar Plexus:

The *Solar Plexus* is situated high in the back of the abdomen, between the waist and breastbone and is a centre for the main network of nerves and ganglia that pass through it. Focus on this area is a major part of many "alternative" therapies, not without good reason. Work on this area will help to tranquilise and balance your entire system. If you are unsure of massage techniques, place your hands palms down and on top of each other, over the area and breathe deeply. Relax and think calming positive thoughts, centering yourself and gently harmonise your whole being.

This area is of particular benefit for self treatment with essential oils. Again, use both hands one on top of the other, right over left, and gently focus positive thoughts on the area, whilst massaging with a suitable blend. Focus on the solar plexus is particularly therapeutic when relaxing in an aromatic bath, the warmth automatically relaxing the area. Breathe deeply, expanding the solar plexus and let the essential oils work their wonders.

Sore Throat: (Also see Laryngitis)
Massage throat and neck areas, in particular the *sternocleido-mastoid muscle*, (the large muscle shown either side of neck when head is turned) with the following:

Sandalwood   13 drops
Clary Sage   12 drops

    Also gargle with Tea Tree as often as possible and from first sign.

    Substitute Tea Tree for Clary Sage when pregnant.

Spots: (See Acne)

Sprains:
A sprain is where the ligament that supports a joint has been damaged. *Never* massage a sprain, but always think *"ICE" - Ice, Compression and Elevation.*

    Use Chamomile and Lavender to reduce inflammation and reduce heat and pain. Place three drops of each in a litre or so of ice cold water. Place a compress over the area and ice on top of that. For speed, unless you happen to have a medical freeze pack, grab a pack of frozen vegetables from the freezer (peas are the easiest to mould to the area), strap that over the compress, and raise the area above the heart if possible. Repeat the compresses as often as possible until you can get to your GP, as it could be a small fracture or involve further complication.

Stiffness: (Also see Massage)
Stiffness is usually due to a lack of mobility and consequent lack of circulation. The most natural method of easing stiffness is to rub the area to bring back some life, so massage away with some toning and rejuvenating essential oils.

    Use: Frankincense, Geranium, Rosemary or Lemongrass, Neroli, Peppermint or Eucalyptus, Bergamot, Black Pepper.

Try

Rosemary	10 drops
Geranium	6 drops
Bergamot	6 drops
Peppermint/Black pepper	2 drops – in 50mls.

If pregnant use:

Petitgrain/Orange	10 drops
Rosewood	8 drops
Geranium	4 drops
Black Pepper	2 drops – in 50mls.

Stings: (See Bites and Stings)

Stomach: (See Abdomen)

Stress:
Our body and its systems can cope wih the majority of what we put it through, sometimes with quite remarkable and miraculous results, but when an imbalance occurs, usually due to an excess, the natural balance and cycle of compensation is disturbed. There is a fine line between natural excitement and stress. Both are a natural experience as we need stimulation, but an excess of healthy tension results in stress, often called the disease of our time.

Stress, and the countless related conditions associated with it, is high on the list of the most prevalent health problems of today. Stress can be any factor which impairs or threatens our health and which has a negative effect on our functioning. Constant or prolonged stress can lead to hormone imbalane, reduced mental and physical performance and diminished immunity and function.

An aromatherapy massage is one of the most effective anti-stress treatments available. Deep relaxation with massage to release tension, combined with the therapeutic benefits of the essential oils has a profound influence on countless stress related conditions.

Being emotionally exhausted, drains our resources and lowers our resistance to illness, illness being common to those more susceptible to stress. Health problems are a common result of our lack of being able to deal with stressful circumstances. If not remedied, a vicious circle of stress, depression, lack of sleep and tiredness, can quickly lead to low immunity, exhaustion and disease. The most important step is to recognise that help is needed, and not to keep on until finally the body says enough is enough - even if you won't.

The word aromatherapy is synonymous with anti-stress and there are countless combinations of suitable oils to sedate, fortify, uplift or relax.

Use:

Bergamot, Neroli, Jasmine, Lavender, Chamomile, Clary Sage, Rose, Frankincense, Sandalwood or Marjoram*. *(If not depressed)

Chamomile/Lavender	10 drops
Clary Sage/Geranium	5 drops
Frankincense/Benzoin	5 drops
Neroli	3 drops

For exhaustive stress, use:

Bergamot	10 drops
Frankincense	8 drops
Rose /Jasmine/Neroli	3 drops

During pregnancy use:

Frankincense	10 drops
Bergamot	6 drops
Neroli/Melissa	3 drops
Benzoin	3 drops

All the above in 50mls.

The symptoms of acute stress (of rapid onset but short duration) such as irritability, tiredness and general aches and pains, are often "eased" by mild stimulants such as more tea or coffee and much sighing. It is at this stage that using the oils with deep relaxation techniques, aromatic baths and early nights, along with fresh air and exercise can prevent the condition progressing. The next stage is reduced immunity, frequent colds and infection, more persistant aches and pains, possible allergies and sensitivities developing, with depression looming.

Stress can be mental, emotional, physical or environmental, and depending on the individual reaction, is often "eased" by taking more stimulants to avoid the issues, frequently leading on to escapism, over drinking, smoking, drugs and worse. Be aware at the outset, and do all you can to change the circumstances. Use the essential oils to balance the system, follow your own personal relaxation techniques and be massaged as often as you possibly can.

Stretch Marks:
Stretch marks may occur anywhere in the body, but commonly on areas more likely to put on weight, such as tops of thighs, buttocks, breasts and of course, abdomen. Being the prime guinea-pig for this book, and having sensitive skin not prone to too much elasticity, I used the following blend everywhere except my right hand breast, which was the only place I marked. (The sacrifices one makes for ones work!) Anyway, it worked for me, and I hope it does the same for you:

Lavender	4 drops
Chamomile	4 drops
Neroli	4 drops
Rose	2 drops

Blend in 30mls of carrier oil, made up of:
90% almond
10% wheatgerm, avocado or jojoba.

Other blends you might like to try include:

Lavender/Chamomile	4 drops
Petitgrain	4 drops
Bergamot	4 drops
Rose	2 drops

or

Lavender/Chamomile	4 drops
Neroli/Rose	4 drops
Frankincense	4 drops
Bergamot	2 drops

To help prevent stretch marks, the massage is important to improve circulation and stimulate the skin. Avoid stimulating massage on the tummy area, but lightly stroke the blend into the skin, loving baby at the same time as yourself. You might also like to add the contents of vitamin E and/or Evening Primrose capsules to the blend.

Sunburn:

Like any burn to the skin, sunburn should be treated seriously, especially as it normally covers a large area. As with all burns, Lavender oil is the first choice, along with Chamomile, to soothe and cool sore skin and to reduce any possible inflammation. With all burns it is essential to reduce the heat in the skin, so bathe in cool water with five drops of each oil added to the water. For more severe burning, add 10 drops of Lavender to a tablespoon of oil and gently smoothe over the affected area, then cover with a tepid compress of Lavender, Chamomile and Tea Tree.

For a nourishing after sun treatment, to soften skin and help preserve the tan, use:

Lavender	12 drops
Chamomile/Bergamot*	6 drops
Rose	2 drops - In 25mls of oil.

*Don't forget to avoid Bergamot oil when going out in the sun, and always use a protective cream, especially on children. If not going into the sun, as it might even be pouring with rain, here is your chance to substitute Bergamot for Chamomile, which will also cheer you up a bit!

Swelling: (See Oedema)

Synergist:

Essential oils work exceptionally well in a *synergistic* blend. This means that one interacts with another to produce greater influence and activity, being greater than if used separately. This is especially so in aromatherapy, when two or more essential oils combined can result in a particular and increased potency. However, never ever think that more is better - because it is not. In aromatherapy, it is the particular combination of the amounts of each oil that has the synergistic effect required. In a volume of 100mls of oil, only one drop of a certain oil can often change a whole blend and its particular influence.

Tachycardia: (Also see Palpitations)

Palpitations are the heart's normal reaction to certain situations, and unless this faster than normal heart beat reduces naturally, once the circumstances have changed (such as after shock or crisis), the condition could be *Tachycardia*, which may lead to serious complication. As always, if in any doubt, seek professional advice, as early medical intervention may be necessary.

Teeth:

On average, the first teeth appear between six months and one year of age. By about three years old, all the first teeth have come through. At about six years of age, the first permanent teeth begin to appear, the new front teeth being easy to see (also lack of them!) but also the larger teeth at the back of the mouth, top and bottom, behind the "baby teeth". These are the ones that we hope will last a lifetime.

Avoid encouraging your child to eat sweet things and cultivating a taste for sugar. Offer some raw carrot, fruit or cheese as a snack between meals. Make a game of brushing teeth together and avoid it being a chore, starting when baby is quite small and can enjoy copying you. Make it a habit she will thank you for, and don't forget to make make friends with your dentist as soon as possible. Regular checkups at the dentist can prevent major traumas later on, and she will probably avoid having anything done whilst there. Get her used to going - and it not being an unpleasant experience, and explain to her why. Essential oils are commonly used in toothpaste.

Teething and Toothache:

When a tooth or teeth are on their way, a child's general resistance may be lowered, and apart from feeling rotten as the process can be painful, she might be susceptible to germs and infection, so do watch her. Avoid the cycle of sleeplessness and anxiety, and anything minor being blamed on teething, she might be feeling no trouble at all from her new teeth, but might have caught an infection.

She might be perfectly fine, one minute without, and the

next with a bright, white new tooth on its way, smiles as well. She could however, be quite distressed, be more than unsettled and have difficulty sleeping; she might have a runny nose and dribble a lot, and this may lead to her urine becoming more acidic and could lead to nappy rash. Try her with "Biccy Pegs", a brand of well established and very effective hard biscuit sold at most chemists, or a freezable teething ring.

Use Chamomile and Lavender equally in 1% dilution (three drops of each in 30mls of carrier oil) and gently stroke the cheeks, jaw line and upper neck with the blend. Treat both sides, as teeth generally come through on both sides within a short time of each other. Homeopathic Chamomile preparations are also excellent in bringing relief from teething problems. See your homeopath or chemist. For acute pain, in a non-pregnant adult, use clove oil from the chemist, or a drop of myrrh, on a plug of cotton wool over the tooth, until the dentist is available.

Temperature:
The average temperature is of 98.4°F or 37°C. Babies have a less efficient temperature control system until they are moving about more, so do be aware of any temperature fluctuations.

There are suitable warming oils which have to be used in low dosage, to promote sweating and thus reduce temperature, but these are particularly strong and should be used with great care, so see a professional. (See Fevers)

Thread Veins:
Thread veins or broken capillaries can be caused by extremes of temperature, smoking or alcohol, or be an hereditary condition, exacerbated by the above.

Vasocontricting oils, which cause the tiny blood vessels to contract and thread veins to diminish, include Chamomile, Cypress, Parsley and Rose. Use with Sandalwood and/or Neroli in a 2% dilution in Peach Kernel oil, morning and evening.

This formula has shown success, although only after regular and prolonged use so do persevere.

Expect results after 6 - 8 weeks if not before, using the formula every day.

Sandalwood   12 drops
Neroli   4 drops
Cypress/Parsley   9 drops

Use in 25mls of carrier oil and smooth gently over area.
Avoid extremes of temperature, alcohol and smoking.

Thrush:

Candida, usually *Candida Albicans*, is a yeast like infection usually occuring in moist areas of the body, such as skin folds, mouth, respiratory tract and vagina, a form even affecting babies bottoms sometimes. When of the mouth or vagina, it is commonly known as *Thrush*. Normal and friendly levels of yeasts and bacteria in the body can be affected by many factors encouraging yeasts to multiply and cause Thrush. Both males and females can be carriers, although symptoms usually occur in females. Both should be treated if infection is present.

In women, Thrush usually affects the vagina and vulva causing itching and a thick, white vaginal discharge. This may be accompanied by soreness and pain in passing urine, along with swelling of the vulva. Thrush needs to be taken seriously, as it can lead to more serious and complex conditions.

Thrush infections are common during pregnancy due to the changes in, and increased levels of, hormones in the system, especially oestrogen, which allows yeasts to grow more easily.

Antibiotics kill off organisms in the body, the friendly ones naturally present in the system, along with the invading yeasts. After a course of antibiotics, Thrush is a common complaint, so if susceptible, and a course of antibiotics is unavoidable, advise your GP of your suceptibility.

Yeasts flourish in warmth and moisture, so avoid manmade fibres next to your skin, including tight trousers. Also avoid perfumed toiletries or anything that may cause irritation to the skin on the vulva. Certain sexually transmitted diseases can cause similar symptoms to Thrush, or there could be more than one infection, so any discharge or itching that you have not had before, or you have any doubt about, should be checked and possible tests made. Clamydia for example, has similar symptoms to Thrush, so do see your GP to rule out any other causes. A doctor will be likely to give you pessaries to be inserted into the vagina, and cream for the uncomfortable itching. If the condition does not rapidly improve using self help treatment, see a professional aroma-therapist, as this condition can be treated very effectively using more specialised methods not suitable for home use.

Use pads rather than tampons during your period.

Patchouli   5 drops

Tea Tree   5 drops in a sitz bath, or sit in a large (ish!) bowl of cold water to which you have added two drops of each of the above.

Other oils to use are combinations of Geranium (circulation and balance), Chamomile (anti-inflammatory), Eucalyptus (anti-bacterial) and Lavender (healing and soothing).

Ticklishness:

Many people are extremely ticklish, especially on the feet. This can often be due to nerves or apprehension, so always be sensitive, but also firm and reassuring. Laugh all together if it helps - laughter is one of the most effective releases of tension and a great healer. It's also a lot of fun!

Tonsilitis: (Also see Laryngitis)

Like the spleen, the lymphatics and thymus, the tonsils form part of our defence system against infection and attack. Removing tonsils along with appendix, used to be almost a matter of course, but now is thankfully much less common. They are there for a reason, and two people I know grew another set of tonsils after removal!

Drink plenty of liquids to flush out the impurities, and also to help soothe your throat. The tonsils may be enlarged, infected and uncomfortable, and small yellow spots may be present. Inhalations are excellent treatment for tonsilitis, as the essential oils reach the very area effectively and efficiently.

Use:

Tea Tree	3 drops
Lemon	2 drops
Sandalwood	1 drop as an inhalation.

Mix up a 2 - 3% blend using the same proportions as above, and massage around the throat and neck area.

Gargle with Tea Tree two drops, in half a glass of warm water. Add a dash of lemon juice and/or honey if you dislike the taste.

Toxoplasmosis:

Toxoplasmosis is a disease common in mammals and birds, which can be transmitted to man via undercooked meat, by direct contact, especially with infected cats, or by contaminated soil. *Congenital Toxoplasmosis* is when a woman is infected during pregnancy, and can be very serious. The mother transmits the disease to her child, which can result in mental retardation and blindness. Outside pregnancy, symptoms appear mild, but it can lead to infection of the lymph nodes if immunity is low. Be extra cautious during pregnancy. In France, testing for Toxoplasmosis is routine, however blood testing for the condition is, at the time of writing, still under consideration by the British government. If you do have pets, ensure they are adequately vaccinated and keep litter trays well out of reach of babies and children and be extra cautious over hygeine.

Tranquilisers;

Although tranquilisers are legally prescribed, they can cause serious dependency, and should be avoided if remotely possible. Hundreds of thousands of people take them and almost as many try desperately hard to get off them. They have been prescribed for even minor ailments such as nausea, sweating, palpitations, sleeplessness or depression, all of which can be effectively treated by aromatherapy and other forms of anti-stress treatment.

As in so many stress related conditions, it is the time, the caring and understanding that has the most profound influence, complementary medicine being highly popular precisely for these reasons. In many cases, it is when a specific cause or symptom cannot be isolated, but there are symptoms of stress that tranquilisers are unfortunately prescribed. Aromatherapy is a viable alternative to tranquilisers and combined with relaxation treatment could prevent years of dependency and frequent distress associated with addiction.

If tranquilisers have been prescribed, and a preference for althernative treatment is made, then do consult with your GP, especially if already on such drugs. The more popular tranquilisers include names such as *Valium*, *Librium* and *Ativan*, to name but three. A sudden reduction could lead to serious and unpleasant withdrawal symptoms. However, if a decision has been made to change treatment, avoid further dependence, as self help, self esteem and self confidence is very important, especially to those that have been dependent for a long time. A commitment has to be made to help oneself, to keep appointments and not expect it to be as "easy" as taking a pill.

At the time of writing there are new antibiotics available to treat depression, in place of the many tranquilisers that cause addiction and distressing side effects. They replace the chemicals lacking in the system that cause depression - which is a recognised medical condition. Always seek professional help, especially if unpleasant side effects are being experienced, and ask to change treatment.

Calming, quietening oils should be used with strengthening and positive oils for maximum therapeutic value.

Lavender	10 drops
Neroli	3 drops
Ylang Ylang	2 drops
Melissa	10 drops
Rose	3 drops
Sandalwood	2 drops
Benzoin	8 drops
G Cham.	5 drops
Clary Sage	2 drops

Blend in 30mls of carrier oil, as massage, on bed linen or in the bath. Carry a few drops on a handkerchief for daily use.

Also see Alcohol for further formulae.

Ultrasound:

Most pregnancies are now monitored by Ultrasound, as an internal picture can be obtained without the use of X-rays. Most parts of the body can be investigated in this way, apart from those covered by bone, or filled with air, such as the lungs. High frequency sound waves are transmitted through the skin and reflected by the internal structures and organs. In pregnancy, the health, age and position of the baby and placenta is easily monitored.

No specific preparation is needed before an ultra-sound test, other than an exceedingly full bladder. This enables the specialist to see the organs more clearly. Hopefully, you will pace this just right. (although it takes some doing), because if your appointment is delayed, there could be a problem...

Clear gel or mineral oil (hopefully warm!), will be smeared on your tummy, as this helps the transmission of the sound waves and for the monitor to slide comfortably over the area. The monitor is a small hand-held transmitter, which is slid over your skin, showing a picture of your baby and womb on a television screen. From this, the specialist can monitor the size of your baby and age, position and health of the placenta, and make various checks to ensure fetal health. It is often possible to have a picture taken from a still of the screen, so it is worthwhile asking. A first for the album! You may be asked to make a donation to the hospital fund, which is certainly worthwhile. The first time I heard my daughter's heart beat nearly floored me, but to see her nestled in my womb, her tiny heart beating away, then turn slightly and raise her arm was indescribable!

The only discomfort if any, is the pressure of the transmit-ter on your by now very full bladder. After a well deserved relief of emptying said bladder, your scan results will hope-fully be discussed with you, or a report sent to your GP. If in

any doubt about *anything* – ask. Further tests may be appropriate, but if it was a routine check to confirm all is well, go
home and be happy, and start "The Album" with your first
photograph.

Umbilical Cord:

Around about when baby is one week old, the "stump"
remaining from the umbilical cord will fall off. The stump has
no nerve supply – you needed no anaesthetic to have it cut at
birth. If the area is a little sore, place one drop of Lavender oil
in one dessertspoonful of oil, mix well and dip a cotton wool
bud in the blend. Gently apply to the area, once each day for a
few days. There should be no complication if the area has
been left alone to let Nature do her work, but has been kept
clean and dry, and if possible, away from the plastic edge of
the nappy. If the area is moist, use a shaped breast pad to
cover it, give protection and to facilitate healing. If swelling or
redness, or indeed any change should occur, always check
with your midwife or GP.

Vaginal Infection:

A vaginal infection is usually known by a yellow or thicker
than usual discharge, this possibly due to the elimination of
infected and waste cells, passing urine could be painful, or
the area may itch and burn and feel most uncomfortable.
Infection could be due to any number of reasons, but as said,
if not usual to you, or you have any doubt whatsoever, seek
professional medical advice.

Varicose Veins:

Varicose veins, like haemorrhoids, are dilated veins. Never
massage directly over varicose veins as further damage could
be caused. Use a compress over the area if possible, or gently
stroke the oil into the skin above the vein, in long even movements in the direction of the heart. Keep feet and legs above
the heart as often as is possible to help with circulation and to
ease pressure. The oils to use are those that are astringent,
diuretic and which have a tonic action on the circulatory
system.

Use if pregnant:

Cypress	5 drops (3)		Geranium	10 drops (3)
Lavender	10 drops (2)	*or*	Cypress/Juniper	8 drops (2)
Geranium	10 drops (1)		Peppermint	4 drops (1)

Use the above in 50 mls of oil, and if using a compress use the figures in brackets to one litre of warm water, alternating with cool.

Verrucas:

A verruca is a plantar wart. They are caused by a virus and usually disappear once resistance has developed. Verrucas are highly contagious and care should be taken in public places, especially public baths where the warm, wet atmosphere is perfect for the virus to establish itself and for infection to spread.

As with athlete's foot, keep the area as clean and dry as possible, always use a separate clean towel (preferably using disposable paper to save on laundry!) and never swap socks, possibly causing "it" to become "them".

Dab a drop of neat Tea Tree on the centre of the spot each day until it disappears, which normally takes a few days.

Vomiting: (See nausea)

Warts:

Warts are caused by a virus and as with verrucas, which are plantar warts, they usually disappear once resistance has developed. There are several types - juvenile warts, found in children and young people; plantar warts as above; common warts, being larger, with a rougher surface and most often on the fingers and hands, and venereal warts, found around the anus and genitals in both sexes.

Warts often occur after shock, trauma or grief, when immunity is low, and usually disappear once general immunity is improved and protection established.

Use one drop of neat Tea Tree on the wart, daily until it disappears.

Water retention: (See Oedema)

Whooping Cough:

Whooping cough is highly infectious, affects mostly children, and can be particularly serious to the under fives. It can lead to pneumonia, collapsed lung, convulsions and even brain damage.

The glottis is normally closed during the cough reflex, and if the child cannot draw enough air in before a cough as is normal, a "whoop" sound results and sudden and violent coughing begins. It is very distressing both for parent and child, as severe and often violent coughing wracks the whole body, often leading to vomiting and extreme anxiety.

If your child has an attack, do try to stay calm, no matter how upset you are. If you aren't calm and reassuring, she will pick up on your panic, which will make it worse, so stay calm and have some Lavender handy to sniff. Don't forget the Rescue Remedy either.

Avoid stuffy, overheated rooms, as this can make the condition worse and further dehydrate. Inhalations and steam can be of great help, and make sure she drinks plenty of liquids, such as fruit juice and water, herb teas and soups.

Use steam inhalations three times per day, to which you have added

Melissa	2 drops
Lavender	1 drop
Eucalyptus	1 drop

Immunisation against whooping cough is now routine, but if you have any reservations, discuss them with informed people you trust.

Worms:

The body is host to many millions of parasites and bacteria, some friendly, some otherwise, and, if you have seen any of the documentaries on the subject, although fascinating, - some absolutely revolting to look at.

Such is the natural flow of things, however this can become a problem when a parasite invades and causes an imbalance in this fine structure and relationship. The most common of worms to inhabit children, is threadworm.

Threadworm is very easily picked up, being very contagious, however any treatment given should be professional. If being treated by a GP or Pharmasist, aromatherapy will not conflict with their treatments.

Use a tummy rub of:

Lavender	3 drops
Roman Chamomile	3 drops
Eucalyptus	3 drops
Tea Tree/Lemon	3 drops - in 50 mls of carrier oil.

As a compress, use one drop of each of the above.

As an inhalation, use:

Fennel	1 drop
Lavender	1 drop
Tea Tree	1 drop

Wounds: (See Accidents)

Zone Therapy: (See Reflexology)

ZZZZZZZZZZZZZZZZZZZZZZZZZZZZZZZZZZZ'ing

Sleep is the most natural cure for everything, a time for healing and giving your body the well deserved rest it needs. Enjoy it!

BIBLIOGRAPHY

W E Arnold-Taylor. Aromatherapy for the Whole Person: Stanley Thornes, Cheltenham, 1991.

Janet Balaskas/Yehudi Gordon. The Ecyclopedia of Pregnancy & Birth: Macdonald & Co Publishers Ltd - London & Sydney 1989.

Arthur & Janet Balaskas. New Life: Sidgwick & Jackson Ltd - London 1979.

John Ball. Understanding Disease: The C. W. Daniel Co Ltd - Essex 1987.

Buchman/Dian Dincin. Herbal Medicine: Rider, London 1991.

Leon Chaitow. Neuro-muscular Technique: Thorsons London 1985.

Mantak Chia. Awaken Healing Energy Through the Tao: Aurora, 1983.

Deepak Chopra. Quantum Healing: Bantam, USA & Canada 1989.

John T Cottingham. Healing Through Touch: The Rolf Institute, Colorado 1987.

Patricia Davis. Aromatherapy an A - Z: The C. W. Daniel Co Ltd, Essex 1989.

Patricia Davis. Subtle Aromatherapy: The C. W. Daniel Co Ltd - Essex 1991.

Dr Stephen Davies & Dr Alan Stewart. Nutritional Medicine: Pan, London 1987.

George Downing. The Massage Book: Penguin Middlesex 1972.

Susan Drury. Tea Tree Oil: The C W Daniel Co Ltd: Essex 1991.

Arlene Eisenberg/Heidi Murkoff/Sandee Hathaway. What to eat when you are expecting: Thorsons London 1986.

Grace Firth. Secrets of the Still: E P M Publications Inc. Virginia, 1983.

Susan Fischer-Rizzi. Complete Aromatherapy Handbook: Sterling Publishing Company: New York 1990.

Ina May Gaskin. Spiritual Midwifery: The Book Publishing Company, Tennessee U.S.A. 1977.

Judy Graham. Evening Primrose Oil: Thorsons Publishing - London, 1984.

Nina Grunfield. Pregnancy Week by Week: Conran Octopus Ltd London 1988.

Felicia Stewart/Gary Stewart/Felicia Guest/Robert Hatcher. My Body My Health: John Wiley and Sons Inc. New York 1979.

Cathy Hopkins. The Joy of Aromatherapy: Angus & Robertson, Australia 1991.

Sally Inch. Birthrights: Hutchinson & Co, London 1982.

Judith Jackson. Aromatherapy: Dorling Kindersley, London 1987.

Leslie Kenton. Ageless Ageing: Arrow Books Ltd, London 1986.

Dr Julian Kenyon. Acupressure Techniques: Thorsons, London 1987.

Sheila Kitzinger. The Experience of Breastfeeding. Penguin Books Ltd, London 1984.

Sheila Kitzinger. The Experience of Childbirth; Penguin Books Ltd, London 1984.

Kevin & Barbara Kunz The Complete Guide to Foot Reflexology: Thorsons, London 1984.

Max Lake. Scents and Sensuality: John Murray Publishers Ltd, London 1989.

Raymond Lautié/André Passebecq. Aromatherapy - The use of Plant Essences in Healing: Chaucer Press, Suffolk 1984.

Donald Law. The Concise Herbal Encyclopedia: Bartholomew & Son Ltd, Edinburgh 1982.

Donald Law. Herb Growing for Health: John Gifford Ltd, London 1975.

Penelope Leach. Baby & Child: Penguin, London 1984.

Claire Loewenfeld/Philippa Back. The Complete Book of Herbs and Spices: David & Charles Publishers Ltd, London 1979

Hanne Marquardt. Reflex Zone Therapy of the Feet: Thorsons London 1983.

Marguerite Maury. Guide to Aromatherapy - The Secret of Life and Youth: The C. W. Daniel & Co Ltd, Essex 1989.

Gill Martin. Alternative Health Aromatherapy: Macdonald & Co, London 1989.

Clare Maxwell-Hudson. The Complete Book of Massage: Dorling Kindesley, London 1988.

Joannah Metcalfe. Culpepper Guide to Herbs and Aromatherapy: Webb & Bower/Penguin Exeter 1989.

Michael McIntyre. Herbal Medicine for Everyone: Arkana, London 1990.

Ashley Montagu. Touching - The Human Significance of the Skin: Harper & Row New York 1986.

Earl Mindell. The Vitamin Bible: Arlington Books, London 1985.

Dr Lila Nachtigal/Joan Rattner Heilman. Oestrogen, The New Women's Dynamic: Arlington Books Ltd, London 1987.

Wataru Ohashi. Do it Yourself Shiatsu: Unwin Paperbacks, London 1979.

Sylvia Klein Olkein. Positive Pregnancy Fitness: Avery Publishing Group, New York 1987.

Jean Palaiseul. Grandmother's Secrets: Penguin 1979.

Earnest Lawrence Rossi. The Psychobiology of Mind-Body Healing: W. W. Norton & Co INc., New York 1986.

Danièle Ryman. Using Essential Oils for Health & Beauty: Century Hutchinson Ltd, London 1986.

Danièle Ryman. The Aromatherapy Handbook: The C. W. Daniel Co Ltd, Essex 1991.

Wanda Sellar. The Directory of Essential Oils: The C. W. Daniel Co Ltd, Essex 1992.

Dr Caroline M Shreeve. The Alternative Dictionary of Symptoms and Cures: Century Hutchinson, London 1989.

John F Thie. Touch for Health: DeVross & Co, California 1979.

William A R Thomson. Healing Plants: MacMillan, London 1980.

Maggie Tisserand. Aromatherapy for Women: Thorsons, London 1985.

Robert Tisserand Aromatherapy for Everyone: Penguin, London 1988.

Robert Tisserand, The Art of Aromatherapy: The C. W. Daniel Co Ltd, Essex 1983.

The Essential Oil Safety Data Manual: The Assoc. of Tisserand Aromatherapists, Brighton.

Steve Van Toller/George Dodd. Perfumery - The Psychology and Biology of Fragrance: Chapman & Hall, London 1988.

Ross Trattler. Better Health Through Natural healing: Thorsons, London 1987.

Dr Jean Valnet. The Practice of Aromatherapy: The C. W. Daniel Co Ltd, Essex 1982.

Patsy Westcott. Alternative Healthcare for Women: Thorsons, London 1987.

Christine Wildwood. Aromatherapy - Massage with Essential Oils: Element Books Ltd, Dorset 1991.

Ross & Wilson. Foundations of Anatomy and Physiology: Churchill Livingstone, New York 1984.

Prof Robert Winston. Infertility - A Sympathetic Approach: Optima, London 1987.

Valerie Ann Worwood. Aromantics: Pan Books, London 1987.

Valerie Ann Worwood. The Fragrant Pharmacy: MacMillan, London 1990.

USEFUL ADDRESSES

Action Against Allergy
31 Abbey Parade
Merton High Street
London SW19 1DG

Active Birth Centre
55 Dartmouth Park Road
London NW5 1SL
071-267-3006

The British Acupuncture Association and Register
34 Alderney Street
London SW1V 4EU
Tel 081 834 1012

Alaskan Flower Essences
1153 Donna Drive
Fairbanks
Alaska 99712
USA

Alcoholics Anonymous
Local office in telephone book
Alcohol Concern:
305 Gray's Inn Road
London WC1X 8QF
Tel 081 833 3471 - For information, publications and access
to a national network of over 40 advice centres.

**The American Society for Phytotherapy and Aromatherapy
International Inc.**
(formerly The American Aromatherapy Association)
P.O. Box 3679
South Pasadena
CA 91031, USA
Tel: 818 457-1742

Aromatherapy Quarterly
5 Ranelagh Avenue
Barnes Village
London SW13 0BY
Fax: 081 392 1691
An independent quarterly journal established in 1983.

Aroma Vera Inc.
33844 S. Robertson Place
Robertson Place
Los Angeles
CA 90034
USA
(Essential oil and product suppliers)

Aromatherapy Organisations Council (A.O.C.)
John Beney (Chairman)
The Berkshire School of Natural Therapy
Conifers
21 Dukes Wood
Crowthorne
Berks RG11 6NF
Tel: 0344 761715

Aromatherapy Products Ltd
The Knoll business Centre
Old Shoreham Road
Hove
Sussex BN3 7GS
Tel: 0273 412139
(E.O.T.A. Registered)

National Association for Holistic Aromatherapy
PO Box 17622
Boulder
Colorado 80308-7622
USA

Association for Breastfeeding Mothers
131 Mayoll Road
London SE26 4HZ
Tel: 071-461-0022

Association for New Approaches to Cancer (ANAC)
c/o Seekers' Trust
Addington Park
Maidstone
Kent ME19 5BL

Association for Post Natal Illness
7 Gowan Avenue
London SW6 6RH

Association of Reflexologists
Slaters
14 Willow End
London N20 8EP

Aura Vision
28308 Seminary Avenue
Oakland
CA 94605
USA
(For photographs of the aura)

Bodytreats Ltd
15 Approach Road
Raynes Park
London SW20 8BA
(Essential oils and products)

Bristol Cancer Help Centre
Grove House
Cornwallis Grove
Clifton
Bristol BS8 4PG

British Reflexology Association
Monks Orchard
Whitbourne
Worcester WR6 5RB

British Acupuncture Association
34 Alderney Street
London SW1V 4EU

British Chiropractic Association
5 First Avenue
Chelmsford
Essex CM1 1RX

British Holistic Medical Association
179 Gloucester Place
London NW1 6DX

British Homoeopathic Association
27a Devonshire Street
London W1N 1RJ

British Herbal Medicine Association
Lane House
Cowling
Keighley
West Yorkshire DB22 OLX

British Migraine Association
178a High Road
Byfleet
Weybridge
Surrey KT14 7ED

British Naturopathic & Osteopathic Association
6 Netherhall Gardens
London NW3 5RR

Child Psychotherapy Trust
The Tavistock Centre
120 Belsize Lane
London NW3 5BA

Childrens' Cancer Help Centre
52 Woodcote Drive
Orpington
Kent BR6 8DB

Cruse
126 Sheen Road
Richmond
Surrey TW9 1UR
(Bereavement counselling and support)

Essential Oil Trade Association (E.O.T.A.)
Gen. Sec. Joe Sapsford
61 Clinton Lane
Kennilworth
Warks CV8 1AS
Tel: 0926 55980   Fax: 0926 512001
(International "watchdog" for maintaining essential oil
quality and funding research).

Food Allergy Association
9 Mill Lane
Shoreham
Sussex

Foresight (Pre-Conceptual care)
Woodhurst
Hydestile
Godalming
Surrey

Institute for Complementary Medicine
21 Portland Place
London W1N 3AF

International Federation of Aromatherapists (I.F.A.)
Department of Continuing Education
Royal Masonic Hospital
Ravenscourt Park
London W6 OTN

International Federation of Reflexologists
78 Eldridge Road
Croydon
Surrey CR0 1SU
Tel: 081 667 9458

International Society of Professional Aromatherapists (I.S.P.A.)
41 Leicester Road
Hinckley
Leics LE10 1LW
Tel: 0455/637987

Both ISPA and the IFA supply details of all qualified aromatherapists that are members, by region and overseas, along with schools and colleges that meet required standards.

The International Journal of Aromatherapy
PO Box 746
Hove
East Sussex BN3 3XA
0273 772479

Institute of Optimum Nutrition
5 Jerdan Place
London SW6 1BE

Kirlian Institute
173 Woburn Towers
Broomcroft Avenue
Northolt UB5 6HU
(Kirlian Photography information/medical use/data)

Ledet Oils
PO Box 2354
Fair Oaks
CA 95628
USA
(Essential oils and products)

Medau Society
8B Robson House
East Street
Epsom
Surrey
Tel: 03727-29056
or
"Tumble Tots" and "Gym Bobs"
Tel: 021-585-7003
(Early exercise benefits for toddlers)

MENCAP
The National Society for the Mentally Handicapped, Children
and Adults:
123 Golden Lane
London EC1 ORT

Miscarriage Association
18 Stoneybrook Close
West Bretton, Wakefield
Yorkshire WS4 4TP

The Multiple Sclerosis Society
25 Effie Road
London SW6 1EE

National Association for the Childless
318 Summer Lane
Birmingham B19 3RL

National Association for PMS
23 Upper Park Road
Kingston Upon Thames
Surrey KT2 5LB

National Autistic Society
276 Willesden Lane
London NW2 5RB

National Childbirth Trust
Alexandra House
Oldham Terrace
London W3 6NH
(N.C.T. classes held nationwide – education for parenthood)

National Federation of Spiritual Healers
Church Street
Sunbury on Thames
Middlesex TW16 6RG

National Institute of Medical Herbalists
41 Hatherley Road
Winchester
Hants SO22 6RR

National Eczema Society
Tavistock House
Tavistock Square
London WC18 9SR

Natural Medicine Society
Regency House
97-107 Hagley Road
Birmingham B16 8BR

New Era Laboratories Ltd
Narfleet
Hull HU9 1BR

Institute of Olfaction
University of Warwick Science Park
Coventry CV4 7AL
Tel: 0203 712014
(Also **Osmotherapy Ltd** at same address)

Pegasus Products Inc.
PO Box 228
Boulder
CO 80306, USA
(California Flower Essences and Gem Elixirs)

Perelandra Ltd
Box 136
Jeffersonstown
VA 22724
USA
(All the Virginian flower essences, rose and garden essences)

Pre-Menstrual Tension Advisory Service
PO Box 268
Hove
East Sussex BN3 1R3

Purple Flame Aromatics
61 Clinton Lane
Kennilworth
Warks CV8 1AS
Tel: 0926 55980 (E.O.T.A. registered)
(Also Purple Flame School of Aromatherapy and Stress
Management)

Quinessence Aromatics
3A Birch Avenue
Whitwick
Leics LE6 3GB
Tel: 0530 38358
(E.O.T.A. registered)

The Raworth Centre
College for Sports Therapy and Natural Medicines
20–26 South Street
Dorking
Surrey RH4 2HQ
Tel: 0306 742150

Royal College of Midwives
15 Mansfield Street
London W1M 0BE
Tel: 071-580-6253

Shirley Price Aromatherapy Ltd
Wesley House
Stockwell Head
Hinckley
Leics LE10 1RD
Tel: 0455 615436   Fax: 0455 615054
(E.O.T.A. registered)

Thursday Plantation Inc
Southcoast Business Park
6440-B Via Real
Carpinteria
California
CA 93013
USA

Thursday Plantation Head Office
Pacific Highway
Ballina
NSW 2378
Australia
(Tea Tree oil suppliers)

The Spastics Society
12 Park Crescent
London W1N 4EQ

U.K.C.C.
23 Portland Place
London W1N 3AF
Tel: 081-637-7181
(United Kingdom Central Council for Nursing, Midwifery and
Health visiting)

The Voluntary Council for Handicapped Children
8 Wakely Street
London EC1V 7QE

INDEX

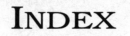

LIST OF OILS
BY PROPERTY

adaptogen oils
Fennel

analgesic oils
Chamomile
Clary Sage
Eucalyptus
Geranium
Lavender
Marjoram
Peppermint
Rosemary

anaphrodisiac oils
Marjoram

anti-bacterial oils
Lemon
Lemongrass
Patchouli
Tea Tree

anti-depressant oils
Clary Sage
Jasmine
Neroli
Orange
Ylang Ylang

anti-fungal oils
Tea Tree

anti-inflammatory oils
Chamomile
Myrrh
Patchouli

anti-spasmodic oils
Basil
Cypress
Fennel
Melissa
Orange
Peppermint

antiseptic oils
Bergamot
Eucalyptus
Garlic
Geranium
Juniper
Lemon
Lemongrass
Myrrh
Patchouli
Sandalwood
Tea Tree

aphrodisiac oils
Clary Sage
Jasmine
Neroli
Patchouli
Rose
Sandalwood
Ylang Ylang

astringent oils
Cypress
Geranium
Lemon

balancing oils
Geranium

calmative oils
Chamomile
Frankincense
Lavender
Neroli
Rose
Ylang Ylang

carminative oils
Lavender
Parsley

cephalic oils
Basil
Peppermint
Rosemary

cleansing oils
Grapefruit
Peppermint

comforting oils
Neroli

cytophylactic oils
Lavender
Neroli
Tea Tree

decongestant oils
Eucalyptus
Fennel
Peppermint

deodorising oils
Bergamot
Clary Sage
Cypress
Eucalyptus
Lavender

Lemongrass
Petitgrain
Rosewood

detoxifying oils
Fennel
Grapefruit
Juniper
Lemon
Rosemary

disinfectant oils
Bergamot
Eucalyptus
Grapefruit
Juniper
Lavender
Lemon
Lemongrass
Tea Tree

diuretic oils
Benzoin
Chamomile
Clary Sage
Cypress
Fennel
Frankincense
Geranium
Juniper
Parsley
Rosemary
Sandalwood

emmenagogue oils
Basil
Chamomile
Clary Sage
Fennel
Geranium
Juniper
Lavender
Marjoram
Myrrh
Peppermint
Rose
Rosemary

euphoric oils
Clary Sage
Jasmine

expectorant oils
Benzoin
Bergamot
Eucalyptus

Lemon
Marjoram
Myrrh
Sandalwood

febrifuge oils
Bergamot Chamomile
Eucalyptus
Lavender
Melissa

fortifying oils
Frankincense
Rosemary

germicide oils
Garlic

haemostatic oils
Geranium
Rose

harmonising oils
Geranium

hypotensive oils
Lemon

oestrogenic oils
Fennel

phototoxic oils
Bergamot

refreshing oils
Basil
Bergamot
Grapefruit
Peppermint
Petitgrain
Rosemary

rejuvenating oils
Frankincense

relaxing oils
Bergamot
Melissa

restorative oils
Basil
Lavender

rubefacient oils
Black Pepper
Cypress

Eucalyptus
Geranium
Juniper
Marjoram
Rosemary

sedative oils
Chamomile
Clary Sage
Lavender
Marjoram
Neroli
Orange
Patchouli
Sandalwood

soothing oils
Chamomile
Frankincense
Sandalwood
Ylang Ylang

spasmodic oils
Fennel

stimulating oils
Basil
Black Pepper
Parsely
Patchouli
Peppermint
Rosemary

strengthening oils
Lemon grass
Patchouli
Rosemary
Sandalwood

toning oils
Basil
Lemon
Lemongrass
Melissa
Parsley
Rose
Rosemary
Rosewood
Sandalwood

toxic oils
Arnica
Basil
Cedarwood
Fennel
Myrrh
Sage
Thuja
Thyme

uplifting oils
Basil
Bergamot
Grapefruit

vasoconstricting oils
Chamomile
Cypress
Parsley
Rose

warming oils
Benzoin
Black Pepper
Marjoram
Patchouli
Peppermint